Copyright © 2020 by Geoffrey Cooling. All rights reserved worldwide. No part of this publication may be replicated, redistributed, or given away in any form without the prior written consent of the author/publisher or the terms relayed to you herein.

Geoffrey Cooling, Hearing Aid Know, 4 Stratton Audley, Bicester, Oxfordshire, OX27 9AU, United Kingdom

If you would like to contact me to ask a question, please don't hesitate to send an email to info@hearingaidknow.com.

Table of Contents

The Dedication 10

Introduction 11

The Year of Bluetooth Customs 15

The Lies We Tell Ourselves..17

Providers of Hearing Aids...23
    Corporate Providers 23
    Independents..26
    Online Hearing Aid Retailers..30
    Shift Hearing Aids & What it Could Mean 33
    Blended Model 33
    What You Need To Know When Buying Online...................................34

Buying a Hearing Aid..41
    Hearing aid price breakdown 42
    Going For the Cheapest Price? 43
    White Label Hearing Aids 44

The Hearing Test..46
    The COSI and Why it is Important 49
    Otoscopy (Examination of the ear)..54
    Case History...54
    Audiometry (Hearing Test) 56
    Speech Testing..59
    Middle Ear Analysis...61
    Tympanometry 61
    Acoustic Reflex Thresholds 62
    Distortion Product Oto-acoustic Emissions (DPOAE)........................63
    Explanation of the results..63
    Hearing Aid Benefit Assessment..63
    Go to the Test Accompanied 64

Understanding Hearing Loss **69**

Conductive Hearing Loss 70

Sensorineural Hearing Loss 71

Mixed Hearing Loss 73

Auditory Processing Disorder 73

The Audiogram 74

Audiogram Markings 76

Hearing Loss Descriptions 77

The Hearing Aids **77**

Hearing Aids, Have Realistic Expectations 78

Knowing What You Want Helps 79

Wireless Accessories 80

Be Sure Of What Are You Buying 80

General Considerations 81

Make Sure You Have a Written Agreement 82

What If Hearing Aids Are Not Enough? **83**

Why Would Hearing Aids Not Help? 83

Speech Discrimination Score 84

Assistive Listening Devices 85

The Multi Mic 86

Personal Experience With Connect Clip 87

Aren't Telecoils Obsolete? 88

Fitting the Hearing Aids **90**

The Fitting 90

Getting Comfortable With Your Hearing Aids 90

The Batteries 91

Controls on Your Hearing Aids 91

Cleaning & Caring For Your Hearing Aids 92

Assistive Listening and Alerting Devices 92

Real Ear Measurements **94**

Why are REMs and Live Speech Mapping Important? 95

The Possible Pitfalls 96

How is it Done?..96

When Should it be Done?..98

The Best Possible Outcome 99

Find A Provider Who Does..100

The Follow-up Visit 101

Fine Tuning 101

Reinforcement of Information...102

Ask Your Questions..102

Telecare 103

Introduction of Telecare by Signia...103

Expansion of Telecare by Resound 103

Complete Real-Time Telecare..103

Face to Face Remote Meetings 104

Why Should You Care?...104

What it Will Do 104

Complete Remote Care 105

Hearing Aid Pricing 105

What Goes Into The Price? 106

Let's Break Down the Price 106

That is Not Justification 107

Changing Prices Internationally 109

A good thing and a bad thing...110

Unbundled pricing 111

Hearing Aid Manufacturers 112

Oticon...113

Oticon Hearing Aids 114

The Platform 116

Opn S Hearing Aid Prices 117

Opn S Hearing Aids 118

Widex 120

Widex Hearing Aids 120

The Platform 121

Widex Moment 121

Widex Moment Hearing Aid Prices 123

Widex Moment Hearing Aids 123

Widex Evoke 126

Widex Evoke Hearing Aid Prices 127

Widex Evoke Hearing Aids 127

Phonak 130

Phonak Hearing Aids 130

The Platform 131

The Roger Pen 136

The Roger Select 136

The Hearing Aids 137

Audeo Marvel Hearing Aids 137

Virto Marvel Hearing Aids 139

Bolero Marvel Hearing Aids 141

Naida Marvel Hearing Aids 142

Starkey 144

Starkey Hearing Aids 144

The Platform 144

Livio Edge 145

Livio Edge AI Hearing Aids 147

Livio AI Hearing Aids 148

SoundLens Synergy IQ 153

Muse IQ 154

The Halo IQ 155

Starkey Technology Levels 156

Signia /Sivantos /Siemens 157

Signia Hearing Aids 157

Telecare 3.0 158

The Platform 158

Signia Xperience 158

Signia Xperience Hearing Aids 161

Signia Nx Hearing Aids 162

GN Resound **167**

Resound Hearing Aids 167

The Platform 167

Linx Quattro Hearing Aids 168

Enzo Quattro Hearing Aids 172

Resound Technology Levels 172

Costco Hearing Aids **173**

Kirkland 9.0 Hearing Aid 173

Kirkland 9.0 Prices 174

The Conclusion 175

Hearing Aid Types, an introduction **177**

Best Advice 177

What Are The Hearing Aid Types? 178

Wireless and Bluetooth Hearing Aids 178

RIC Receiver in Canal Hearing Aids **180**

THE PROS & CONS OF RIC HEARING AIDS 181

Contra-indications To Wearing RICs / RITEs 184

In Finishing 184

ITE In The Ear Hearing Aids **185**

Invisible Hearing Aids 186

The pros and cons of invisible hearing instruments 190

Completely In Canal Hearing Aids / Mini In Canal 191

Full Shell & Half Shell Hearing Aids 192

THE PROS & CONS OF CUSTOM HEARING AIDS 192

Contra-indications To Wearing Custom Hearing Aids 195

In Finishing 195

BTE Behind The Ear Hearing Aids **196**

THE PROS & CONS OF BTE HEARING AIDS 197

Contra-indications To Wearing BTEs 199

Bluetooth / Made For iPhone Hearing Aids **200**
The Problem with Bluetooth 201

Made For Any Phone Hearing Aids **201**
Hands-Free Calls 201
Stereo Streaming 202
Power Hungry 202

Made For Android **202**

Rechargeable Hearing Aids **203**
Why Should You Consider Rechargeable Hearing Aids?...........205
All types of hearing aids?..206
Phonak Rechargeable 207
Signia Rechargeable Hearing Aids 208
Oticon Rechargeable Digital Hearing Aids 209
Resound Rechargeable Digital Hearing Aids.........................209
Starkey Rechargeable Digital Hearing Aids...........................209
Unitron Rechargeable Digital Hearing Aids 209
Widex Rechargeable Digital Hearing Aids.............................210
What Are The Pros and Cons of Rechargeable Hearing Aids? 210
Lithium-ion Rechargeable hearing aids 210
The Cons of Lithium-Ion Rechargeable Hearing Aids..............211
The Pros of Lithium-Ion Rechargeable Hearing Aids 212

Hearing Aid Technology Levels **213**
LET'S TALK HEARING AID TECHNOLOGY 213
The Life of a Hearing Aid..213
How Hearing Aids Work..215
Basic technology hearing aids 216
Lifestyle help from basic hearing aid technology 216
Standard technology hearing aids 217
Lifestyle help from standard hearing aid technology 218
Advanced technology hearing aids......................................218

Lifestyle help from advanced hearing aid technology 219

Premium level hearing aids 220

Lifestyle help from premium hearing aids 221

Hearing Aid Features 222

Let's Talk Hearing Aid Features 222

What are the real-world benefits of hearing aid features? 223

Audible indicators in hearing aids 223

Listening programmes in hearing aids 224

Automatic programmes in hearing aids 225

Binaural synchronisation 226

Binaural Compression 227

Compression channels 228

Data logging 229

Feedback cancellation in hearing aids 230

Adaptive feedback cancellation 231

Directional microphones 231

Adaptive directional microphones 232

Automatic directional microphones 232

Frequency bands in hearing aids 233

Hearing aid noise reduction 235

Speech enhancement 236

Transient noise reduction 236

Wind noise reduction 236

Over the Counter Hearing Aids 237

A Greedy Monopoly 238

Are We Greedy? 238

What will it Mean For You 241

Not for Everyone 241

The Freedom to Mess it up 242

What about Traditional Manufacturers? 243

What Will Be Your Experience? 244

Care of the Devices 244

Making the Right Choice 245

Freedom 245

Clean and Care of Hearing Aids **245**

Avoid hearing aid repairs...246

Hearing Aid Care and Maintenance.......................................247

Cleaning of hearing aids and cleaning tools 247

When do wax guards need to be changed? 248

Cleaning and maintenance of an ITE and RIC hearing aid 248

Cleaning & Maintenance of BTE hearing aids........................250

Drying out hearing aids..252

Hearing aid dryers 252

Hearing aid drying cups and tablets 252

Electronic hearing aid dryers 253

In Finishing **255**

The Dedication

To My Dad, Who taught me this:

At the end when your worth is measured, when they talk of your worth. Your worth as a person

it will not be the currency you have earned, the holidays you have taken, the cars you have driven. The house you live in

Your worth, your true worth, that's measured in the life's you have touched. The people you have supported. The people you have defended. The people who you have not let stand alone

The joy you have brought. The lives you have improved. The love you have shared.

The simple human kindness

Because when it comes to that day. These are the things that will be remembered. These are the things that will be your legacy.

If we but remembered this. If we but felt it as truth. Really felt it. Your world. My world. Our world. Would be better

To my father, thank you for the lessons

Introduction

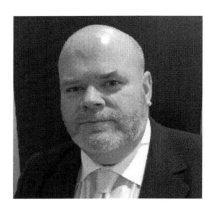

Privately provided hearing aids are a significant investment. I want to give you the knowledge to make that investment with confidence.

I wrote this book initially because I wanted to make sure that there was a good, impartial source of information available to people.

It is precisely the same reason I got involved with the website Hearing Aid Know. In this book, I have again updated the information given and expanded it to include some of the latest developments.

As I sit here writing this year's book I am all too aware of the by now notorious Covid 19 virus and the advent of its arrival on the island of Ireland. Let me explain why, I am 50; I have asthma, I continue to insist on smoking (yes I know, gobshite). All of this means that there is a chance that this may be the very last little book I write.

So, I decided to try and ensure that this is the definitive book, covering every single thing I can think of that any prospective hearing aid user should know. I hope I have done so; I also hope I get to update this book as always later in the year. If not, I want to thank you for buying this book and supporting my family when I can no longer.

My background is relatively simple, I have been involved with hearing aids for close to fifteen years, and they continue to fascinate me. I was a qualified hearing aid audiologist in private practice in Ireland, before moving to work for a major hearing aid manufacturer. I am now back in private practice, operating in Dublin, Ireland.

I collaborate with a guy named Steve Claridge on the website, Hearing Aid Know. We want to bring clear, honest advice to consumers centred on hearing aids and the people who provide them. I like to talk straight, laugh at gobshites (Irish technical term), and my sense of humour may well get on top of me. However, bear with me, and I am usually able to translate the gobbledygook.

What follows is a relatively high-level look at hearing aids, their technology levels, their pros and cons and the features inside. I hope that this will give you the complete grounding in the subject that you need to make educated decisions. In one review of this book, they said that I don't make a comparison of hearing aid brands.

I don't; it would make the book about a thousand pages long. I see my job in this book to give you a high-level understanding of what should matter to you. I also try to make sure I at least touch on the latest and best hearing aids from the major manufacturers. Without actually physically seeing you, I can't make a comparison and recommend the best for you. It is just impossible.

All I will say is that each of the major hearing aid brands offers relatively outstanding hearing aids that do what they are supposed to. Where I have tried hearing aids (I have a moderate high-frequency hearing loss), I will talk about my experiences.

In one of the reviews given for one of the books somebody said I was encouraging people to go to Audiologists. In the UK and Ireland, we don't have the same set up as in the US. We are all Hearing Aid Audiologists. There are no Hearing Instrument Specialists and Doctors of Audiology here. So while I might have mentioned Audiologists in the text, it wasn't meant to be a recommendation to see an Audiologist in the states.

My feeling, in general, is that you should go to the person who has excellent reviews, no matter what their level of qualification. In my experience, I have seen Hearing Aid Audiologists, Hearing Instrument Dispensers and Doctors of Audiology who were halfwits whom I wouldn't let treat my dog.

So the level of education is no guarantee of efficacy. The biggest question you should ask any hearing care professional is, do they undertake Real Ear Measurements or Speech Mapping of hearing aids. If they say no, tell them you will go somewhere else that does.

You can read more about hearing aids and the people who provide them on our website at Hearing Aid Know

The Year of Bluetooth Customs

2020 is very young, but it already seems like it is going to be the year of Bluetooth In The Ear Hearing Aids. Resound finished 2019 with the new LiNX Quattro Bluetooth custom hearing aids.

They will connect to iPhones and compatible Android phones for both streaming audio and phone calls. One of the new Quattro customs is the first-ever Bluetooth, direct connection CIC. In fairness to everyone, in general, it is a little larger than a CIC. Nonetheless, they managed to pack direct connection into a tiny package.

Already in 2020, we have seen Phonak introduce the Virto Black device at CES, which is a Marvel In The Ear hearing aid. That means direct connection to any Bluetooth enabled phone, Android, iPhones, even so-called dumbphones all in an In The Canal or maybe half-shell size hearing aid.

Starkey quickly followed with the introduction of their new Edge platform that has the first-ever lithium-ion rechargeable Bluetooth custom hearing aid. The devices will connect to iPhones and compatible Android phones for streaming audio and taking phone calls.

The Starkey Edge is genuinely a breakthrough device, but we will talk about that later in the book. What it all adds up to is an exciting year for Bluetooth In The Ear hearing aids.

I would imagine that all of the rest of the hearing aid brands will be upgrading their custom hearing aids this year and considering the direct connection to compatible Android phones. Although, with the new Bluetooth standard coming to a device near you in 2020 or 2021, it is hard to know. No matter what the other brands do, I think that 2020 will be the year for choice in this segment of the market.

The Lies We Tell Ourselves

Hearing loss happens; the best thing to do is deal with it. I wrote on the Hearing Aid Know site about the lies we tell ourselves about why we don't need hearing aids, and I want to detail them here.

My Hearing Loss isn't Severe Enough

Hell no! Your wife or husband is about to strangle your ass. If she or he has to repeat themselves one more time she will happily kick you until your unconscious, unconscious I tell you!

Even a Mild Hearing Loss

Apart from your wife or husband harbouring homicidal thoughts, we now know that we need to treat even a mild hearing loss. Recent evidence that has come to light about untreated hearing loss and cognitive decline frightened me so much I started wearing my hearing aids all the time.

Hearing Loss & Cognitive Decline

Let me explain, we as professionals were always worried about the broader effect of hearing loss on general health and emotional well-being. In the last few years, though, evidence has come to light that connects untreated hearing loss to more rapid cognitive decline and possibly dementia.

The evidence has made us as professionals change our thoughts about intervention in hearing loss. We are now recommending hearing aids even for mild hearing losses that we may not have before.

So, it's pretty simple; if you have a hearing loss at all, you should think about treating it with hearing aids if they are appropriate.

Hearing Aids are Uncomfortable

Yes, that's right; they are strange at the beginning. You have never worn something in your ear all day before. Why in hell would they not be uncomfortable or foreign?

That feeling will fade with a little time. If it hasn't disappeared in a week, you may need to be re-sized. Generally, it is a simple process. Stop using excuses because you don't like the idea of wearing hearing aids. It's time to get over yourself, which brings us to.

I would be Embarrassed to Wear a Hearing Aid

So, I understand that actually, I don't feel it, but I do appreciate it. For me, it is a simple equation, need hearing aids, gets them. I don't give a toss what other people think; in fact, I am probably famous for it.

But, I do understand that other people don't see it as that simple for them. They see having to wear a hearing aid as some sort of statement on them, the ageing process and their worth.

That's all arse (Irish technical term) complete and utter arse. A hearing loss is not a statement on you, on who you are, or how old you are; it merely is.

No more and no less. It is a problem that is causing you real issues. Not doing something about a hearing loss that is affecting your life, now that is a statement about you.

Honestly, is it more embarrassing to be in control of your ability to communicate or to stumble through life trying to bluff something while everyone knows you have a problem? Because believe me, everyone knows you have a problem.

Exactly What You Are Missing

Let's think about this: what are you missing, what are you losing out on by not dealing with your hearing loss? The whispered words of a loved one, the pure joy of a particularly moving piece of music, the soft voices of your Grandchildren, the pleasure of easy social contact.

So much of the joys of life are based on communication and engagement. Robbing yourself of the ability to be genuinely involved is just damn stupid. Are you stupid? You are reading this book, so I imagine you probably aren't.

The Joy of Easy Communication

How much do you miss the joy of easy communication, getting the joke first time, instead of them having to repeat themselves?

The frustration of having to ask someone "what did they say?" The sitting in a room of people you love while being almost completely isolated. The simple joy of easy conversation.

You know the next time you are tired and worn out from the effort needed to listen? Do you know that feeling of stress, that feeling of being overwhelmed?

You know the simmering strife in your home life because the people you love are at their wits end? Well, you can quickly deal with most of that by using hearing aids.

Damn it, Reclaim Your Life!

Reclaim your life, it is as simple as that, are you ready to pack up and die? Well if you aren't, get on with living.

I do not want to admit a hearing loss in public

Why? I go back to my last statement; everyone knows you have a hearing loss. Believe me; they knew long before you did. So why are you anxious?

You are concerned about being embarrassed, but believe me, and you know it well. You will be more embarrassed by getting everything wrong, asking people to repeat themselves and generally looking like you are doddering a bit.

Yup, doddering! Let me ask you this, which looks older and a little senile? A person who seems to be always forgetful, who asks others several times to repeat themselves, gives the wrong answers to questions, always confuses words and continually goes on about how people didn't mumble so much in my day.

Or, someone who takes control of their ability to communicate lives an active social life and is generally happier with their lives? Think about that; I know what the right answer is, and so do you.

Hearing Aids Do Not Work in Noisy Environments

Yes, they do, especially if you buy the right level of technology for you. Simply put, if you want to hear well in complex sound situations, you need to think about the top two tiers of hearing aid technology.

Does that mean that the bottom two levels of technology won't help you? No, it doesn't, they will help you a great deal, especially if you use something like a remote mic to give you an extra bit of help.

Hearing aids will work to provide you with the sound cues you need to understand what people are saying. Will they allow you to hear everything in a complex, noisy situation? Maybe not, but you have to realise that even people with perfect hearing have problems with noise sometimes.

The key to being happy with your hearing aid purchase is to be realistic about what you should hear with them. You need to be realistic about your expectations of the hearing aids you buy as well. A competent professional should guide you on this; they should try to make it clear what to expect from the hearing aids.

I Have More Serious Priorities

You probably don't, back to what I was talking about earlier. Our new understanding of the effects of hearing loss on general health and cognitive function makes treating hearing loss a priority. As I said, we have changed how we think, and we are recommending the treatment of even mild hearing loss.

I do understand that there may be other things going on in your life, things that make it challenging to consider your ability to hear as a priority for you. But your ability to hear and understand is your ability to communicate with ease. That affects all the different parts of your life.

They don't Restore Your Hearing to Normal

I am afraid nothing can restore your hearing to normal, but hearing aids do a damn good job at giving you normal levels of hearing. They are the difference between hearing what is being said and saying what? All the time. They will allow you to communicate freely and easily.

I Hear Well Enough in Most Situations

Yes, about that, nope. Ask your long-suffering family about that. People often say to me "I hear well in one to one situations". Generally, people with hearing loss do okay in one to one situations where their companion is facing them, and the face is well lit. With no competing noise and full view of the person's face, they get on okay.

However, we do a simple speech test with many people, words presented at normal speech levels. Of course, there are no visual references, so they are relying on their hearing only. When they have gotten three out of five or six out of ten words wrong, they suddenly realise they aren't doing as well as they thought they were.

Damn it be a grown-up

Yup, enough prevaricating, enough lying to yourself, enough excuses. You owe it to yourself and your ongoing health and happiness. Hell, you owe it to your long-suffering family. Time to put your big boy or big girl pants on. This is too important to hide behind bull, believe me when I say it. Hearing loss isn't a statement of who you are, not getting proper treatment for it and trying to bluff is.

Providers of Hearing Aids

To privately procure a hearing aid, you need to attend a provider, pretty simple. However, you have a choice of different types of providers available to you. That choice has grown in recent years beyond the two traditional outlet types, which were large corporate businesses and independent businesses.

There are corporate type providers such as Amplifon, Hidden Hearing, Boots and Specsavers in the UK and Miracle-Ear, Hear USA, Costco and Beltone in the US.

Independent providers may be sizeable multiple branch outlets or smaller single outlet businesses.

In the recent past, we have seen another type of provider arrive, the Online Provider. They offer savings based on the fact that they have no shop front and small overheads.

In the next few pages, I would like to explore these outlet types and explain the pros and cons of each one of these very different provider types.

Corporate Providers

In my experience, Corporate providers generally offer a pretty good service including on-going aftercare, although with many the experience can be a bit like being on a conveyor belt.

I worked for Amplifon in Ireland back in the day, and I have to say that they were on the cutting edge of best practice and service. We provided an outstanding level of service to our Patients, and they still do.

However, we worked within the constraints that were set, and our business was sales. Don't get me wrong, it also involved real committed care, but sales were what it was all about. Most corporate providers are built on this system; there is always some pressure on staff to sell, which is how they survive.

That isn't necessarily a bad thing, yes they are trying to sell you hearing aids but believe me they won't try, if you don't need them. Knowing the core ethos of that company, I can think of worse people to buy a hearing aid from.

Pressure To Sell Specific Products

There will usually be some pressure on staff to sell one product line specifically in most corporate chains. Again Amplifon was a little different, they have a wide selection of brands, but the pricing of the devices tends to control what is sold.

Amplifon is a corporate entity, but it is, in fact, independent of any manufacturer, as is Costco in the states. There are very few genuinely Independent corporate retail organisations in hearing care.

Arrangements with Manufacturers

They have agreements with particular manufacturers, and those arrangements mean that certain brands are more advantageous for them to sell. However, as long as I was in Amplifon, Corporate Management didn't interfere at the macro level. They allowed Dispensers to sell whatever they felt was best for the patient in front of them.

Owned By Hearing Aid Manufacturers

Many corporate providers are owned by hearing aid manufacturers. While some of them may have different hearing aid brands on their price lists, they are more likely to sell you the brand that owns them. The fact that a business is owned or part-owned by a hearing aid brand is very rarely obvious or publicised.

For instance, Boots Hearing Care in the UK is part-owned by Sonova, the owners of the Phonak and Unitron hearing aid brands. In the US, Sonova also owns Connect Hearing. William Demant, the owners of the Oticon and Bernafon brands, own Hidden Hearing (another UK company).

GN Resound owns Beltone in the US. It isn't just these hearing aid brands; every major hearing aid brand has some retail arm. This type of vertical integration is only increasing within the business; more and more manufacturers are buying retail outlets.

Limiting of Choice?

I believe that this vertical integration limits your choices, the equation is simple, and more often than not, you are getting one brand no matter what. Honestly, this doesn't necessarily mean that the device or brand won't be suitable for you; it just means there is no real choice on offer.

It isn't that I think that is a bad thing; I feel that you should be clear on it. The business really should make it clear to you; I believe an educated decision is nearly always a good one.

In essence, while corporates try to ensure that the best service and experience is on offer across their chains, it is sometimes not the case. The standard of care can still vary, just as the standard of care provided by Independents can vary.

Another problem with Corporates is that there can be a good bit of staff turnover so you may buy from one person, but end up being seen by another at a later date.

I know that some people find that off-putting, they like to stay with the person they trust, especially if they have built up a relationship with them. However, the fact that Corporates have multiple branches and staff can also be a pro.

If for instance, you are travelling in the UK or across the US, if your provider has an outlet wherever you are, they will see you as a customer if you get in trouble with your hearing aids.

It is also worth considering that if you have issues with the person who supplied you with the hearing aids, there are also other staff members to take care of you. These things do happen, and I have seen them happen many times.

So there are pros and cons to dealing with a corporate entity, just as there are pros and cons to everything.

Independents

Independent providers are just that, independent of any hearing aid manufacturer or corporate entity. They are usually small family-run businesses, although some may be multi-branch.

More often than not though, they are single branch entities that may offer their service in branch and perhaps across a few clinics situated in associated health partners such as Opticians or even Chemists/Pharmacies/Medical Centres.

Access to All Products

Independents generally have access to all of the big hearing aid manufacturers; however, in practice, they will usually only use perhaps three brands at most. There will be a primary brand that they deal with and two secondary brands.

Generally, they pick brands for a variety of reasons, some commercial such as pricing, and some clinical, such as the efficacy of devices and perhaps specialisation.

I have said before, that if I were running an Independent practice, I would probably choose Widex, Phonak and GN Resound as my three suppliers. However, that decision has become harder for me.

Since I first said that, both Oticon and Signia had introduced technology that interests me. So my choice of brands would be a little harder now.

I would try to choose the brands that are able to provide me with pretty much everything I needed to meet the needs of my customers as they presented to me. However, as different innovations came along, I would be considering other brands or re-considering what share of each brand I supplied.

Freedom to Offer Best Service

That is the freedom that being independent delivers; you make the best decisions based on the customer in front of you and the latest and best technology available. I think that is the best way to serve the customer, and indeed, the best option for the customer.

Local Business

Most Independents are local businesses; they often live local to the community they serve. They are usually from your locality that keeps the money in your area. More than that, you know with whom you are doing business. You might not have known them personally, but there was always word of mouth through the community.

Service Instead of Advertising Budget

Independent businesses tend not to have massive marketing budgets. They build their success on service and good word of mouth. They don't survive unless there are both. Independent professionals usually rely on the word of mouth of their customers to succeed in business.

The simple fact is that if they don't treat people right, they don't eat. That is a pretty big incentive. However, more often than not, they are genuinely caring and committed to offering the very best service.

Often Higher Levels of Care

Independent hearing aid providers offer high levels of service and aftercare as standard. They usually have set up their businesses so that they can do just that. National hearing aid providers are getting better and better at looking after their customers. However, everything within those providers is usually to a rigid plan.

Independents are genuinely flexible in their approach, delivering the service and aftercare that is needed when it is required. You probably won't find many others who are as committed to ensuring you have the best experience.

On top of that commitment and because a hearing aid provider is Independent, he or she does not have to march to the company guidelines when it comes to providing hearing aids.

It means that they will recommend hearing aids that are right for you and your lifestyle needs. Hearing healthcare professionals in National businesses will always try to do the same. Inevitably though, because of company policies and changing commercial arrangements, they may have to do so within a limited choice.

Of course, those are all pros, but what about the cons of dealing with Independents? If it is a one-person show, there could be issues with continuity of service. God forbid he or she gets sick, is injured or dies, who will continue to look after you?

If you have issues with your devices while you are travelling, will you have access to help? That depends, if the problem is with the failure of your hearing aid, then you will probably be able to get it fixed under your warranty elsewhere.

Your International Warranty will cover you for such repairs during the warranty period. However, there may well be a handling charge for it. After all, you aren't a customer of the

Practice that is organising the repair and post, and packaging needs to be covered.

For anything else, such as diagnosis of issues, adjustments, wax traps, batteries etc. You will have to pay or negotiate a local price.

Online Hearing Aid Retailers

In recent years there has been an explosion in online hearing aid providers. Initially, the online providers were, in fact, little more than lead generation sites. Their only business was to get your name and address and sell it on to a company local to you. While that model still exists, there has been a divergence in the space in the recent past.

Buying a Hearing Aid Online

The sales of hearing devices online are not new; there are businesses around the world that sell hearing aids online direct to consumers. Some of those businesses do an excellent job of it, in the main because they have that infrastructure in place to ensure the buyer's success.

That infrastructure involves remote testing of the buyer's hearing and remote fitting and fine-tuning of the devices. However, that is not the case with all online hearing aid retailers. Some of the new online retailers are offering hearing aids from the big hearing aid brands.

The infrastructure to support these hearing aids remotely was not there. The manufacturers didn't design these devices to be sold online. However, with the rise of remote support, or tele-audiology, that is changing.

Even with the ability to connect to your hearing aids remotely and fine-tune or fit them, there are still some concerns that I feel I should address.

First, let's talk about online retailers. There are now three types of online hearing aid retailers, they are

Lead Generation Sites

Co-operative Groups

Online Hearing Aid Retailers

The lead generation sites don't need much description; they are merely there to attract you to them, get your name and address and then sell it on to someone in your area. The others are a little interesting and work differently.

Co-Operative Groups
Co-operative groups have mostly spawned from the lead generation sites. They are in essence a group of hearing aid businesses (usually Independents) who are co-operating to drive a website which brings in business.

There is centralised control of the website, which sends enquiries to the nearest hearing healthcare professional in your area. This type of set-up is a traditional model that is using the power of the internet.

Online Hearing Aid Retailers

There are now several pure online hearing aid retailers, some of them such as Blamey & Saunders, MD Hearing Aids or Eargo manufacture hearing aids and sell them online to the public. Some, however, such as Lively Hearing, sell hearing aids from the big six hearing aid brands.

These types of business usually do not have a network of Audiologists that they work with, although, that is beginning to change. I don't think online sales of hearing aids are a terrible thing when there is an infrastructure set up to cater for it.

By that, I mean that online sales are supported by a testing and fitting infrastructure either online or offline. For instance, Blamey and Saunders in Australia deliver a system I support, as does iHear and Eargo in the US.

These companies have purposely set themselves up and designed their technology to offer hearing devices online. The support and infrastructure to provide it are there.

Up to recently, I would not support the sale of hearing aids from the big brands in an online manner mainly because they have not designed them for purchase in that manner. The underlying technology to do this well with the leading hearing aid manufacturers just wasn't there.

That has begun to change, more and more of the hearing aid brands offer remote care systems—basically telecare systems which allow remote fine-tuning of hearing aids. Looking after someone remotely has become far more manageable. Therefore,

I now believe that online sales of main brand hearing aids can make sense in some circumstances.

With the involvement of Sonova (the manufacturer of Phonak, Unitron, AudioNova and Hansaton hearing aids) in Blamey Saunders in Australia and the recent introduction of their **Shift hearing aids**, I think the game is changing.

Shift Hearing Aids & What it Could Mean

Sonova purchased Blamey Saunders outright in 2019. Since the purchase, they have introduced a new model of hearing aids designed to be sold directly to the consumer.

The devices use their Sword chip, the same chipset that powers the Phonak Marvel, Unitron Discover and other devices. The Sword chip gives them full Bluetooth connectivity and access to their remote care system.

They designed Shift Hearing aids to be self-fitting. You purchase the hearing aids online, and when they come, you programme them yourself using an app-based hearing test.

If you need support moving forward, the Blamey Saunders team will offer that support remotely to you. I would imagine that if you need in-person assistance, you will be able to attend one of Blamey Saunders physical locations.

Blended Model

The model they are offering is a blended model. It blends remote care with in-person care, and I think that many of the hearing aid brands could see it as a future model.

I think if you are committed to buying online, this type of model may be the best one for you. I also believe that this type of model is probably going to go global in one way or other over the next five years.

As I said, I am not against buying online. There are, of course, caveats, let's look at them.

What You Need To Know When Buying Online

So here it is, this is what you need to consider when buying online, and the first and most important thing is you need a proper hearing test.

We must base any hearing aid fitting on a reliable hearing test. To ensure a reliable hearing test, we need to be sure the ear canals are clear. In the traditional model, a professional looks in the ear before they undertake a hearing test.

Who is Looking in Your Ears?

If you purchase the hearing aids online, who is looking in your ears? That worries me, how will you know your ears aren't blocked or that there is not some sort of medical problem with your eardrum?

How Will You Identify Medical Problems?

A full hearing test will identify any underlying medical problems that may need further investigation. Most acquired hearing loss is run of the mill sensorineural hearing loss. Without an in-depth hearing test, how will you be sure that there are no grounds for further investigation?

The self-testing process that is offered by many of the online vendors is a simple air-conduction pure-tone hearing test. That isn't enough to identify all referral issues.

In my experience, even when I spoof a referral issue by making one ear far worse than the other, the software does not notify me that I need further investigation. It should, and I hope that all of these vendors are working towards that.

What About Long Term Care?

Hearing aids are not like glasses. You don't just put them on, and everything is lovely. It doesn't work like that, unfortunately. You will need ongoing care and attention to get the very best out of your hearing aids for as long as you have them.

That may well be up to eight to ten years. If you feel confident that the online retailer can give you that care and service and is committed to doing so, then you are onto a winner.

It is both my experience and the experience of Steve that to get on well with hearing aids people generally need the involvement of a good hearing healthcare professional.

We have said it here before, our worry about buying hearing aids online was that people might buy the hearing devices and then find it difficult to get a professional to help them if they need it.

While telecare is pretty good, it isn't going to solve every problem that may arise. So there are several things you need to consider so you can make an educated choice before buying.

What You Need To Think About When Buying a Hearing Aid Online

- You need an in-depth hearing test

- Self-test systems don't offer all the answers

- Hearing aids aren't glasses; they don't just work

- You will need ongoing care

- How will you understand what the best hearing aids for you are?

- Will someone make a recommendation on the best hearing aids for you?

- Will someone fit them for you?

- If You buy them online with no service, how much will the hearing test and fitting cost?

- How much will it cost for aftercare visits or telecare visits? (you are going to need them)

- How much will it cost for repairs?

- How will they handle repairs?

- Finally and the big one, will the extra costs of getting someone local to help you mean a net saving or loss for you?

It struck me that the question I should answer is "Would I be happy to sell you hearing aids online?" That is the real test. So I should answer it, I would be happy to sell you a hearing aid online if, and it's a big if, either the hearing aid manufacturers made the technology available that allowed me to do an in-depth hearing test. Or you had a thorough hearing test undertaken

That the hearing aid brands software allowed me to do a full fitting and verification of the hearing aids remotely and finally and probably most importantly, that I was confident that you were able and tech-savvy.

Those conditions are not nearly as far from existing as they once were. To be honest, if I thought you could manage well and if you were able to supply me with in-depth testing results, I probably would consider selling you a hearing aid from one of the prominent manufacturers online, but I would warn you that I could not do real ear measurements which I feel are vital.

That is a big statement coming from me. Up to recently, I would not have considered doing so. I would still be cautious about doing it, but I am more willing to do so now.

As I said, I would still be worried about Real Ear Measurements (something that we will discuss later). I can't do them remotely, and may not ever be able to. That is still a stumbling block for me.

What does it Matter to You?

First of all, you want the latest and best for you and your hearing loss; it is as simple as that. Secondly, hearing aids aren't the same as glasses. You do not just put them on, and everything is fine. That is a simple truth, hearing aids take time to get used to, and to get the best out of them takes time.

You might not realise it, but the services of a good hearing professional are imperative to your ongoing experience. For you to get the best out of any hearing aids you buy; you will need a committed and skilful professional to help you.

Why do You Need Help?

As I said, hearing aids are not like glasses; firstly, by the time you choose to buy hearing aids, you will probably have been suffering a hearing loss for up to seven years or more.

If I were to give you full amplification (the prescription you needed to correct your hearing), you would run screaming from my office. You wouldn't like it one bit; you would find the level of amplification overwhelming.

So, I will first set you to a reduced prescription, one that benefits you but doesn't challenge you too much. You will still note a dramatic difference. However, it will be as much as you can handle. Over time, which varies from customer to customer, I will then increase the amplification to your prescription level.

Not every Professional will follow this protocol. Modern hearing aids have an auto-acclimatisation feature. It is a feature that I can set, at the first fitting, which will gently turn the hearing aid prescription up towards your prescription level over a controllable and customisable level of time.

I use the system; however, I still like to see the customer during this period to assess the increase and to discuss the changes and their experiences. I believe that this is the best way to serve my customers.

We base your prescription on your hearing loss. Thousands of hours of research on thousands of ears has gone into that prescription. It is an excellent starting point. However, everyone is different. I have found that most people need further personalisation of their amplification to get the best out of their hearing aids.

So, with that in mind, even when you get to your prescription level, which I will validate with Speech Mapping (more about that later). You still need some tweaking. I think this makes the situation a bit clearer, and it is why you can't compare hearing aids to glasses, or perhaps any other device. Let's talk about customisation of sound.

Think it's Over Then? Think Again

As I said, the prescription isn't when the fat lady sings. Generally, your prescription level is just a starting point, a good starting point but merely a starting point.

Hearing is a very personal sense, and appreciation of sound differs. I like classical music, and my wife thinks it is noise. Each one of us is slightly different, unique. Most people will need some fine-tuning undertaken around their prescription to be happy with the sound of their hearing aids.

So finally, after all those appointments we have got you to a place where the sound the hearing aids produce is just right for you. That's when we start investigating the settings for different situations and discussing how you are getting on generally.

The rehabilitation process doesn't happen in the first week or month; it takes time and effort both on your part and the part of the professional who is helping you. That professional needs to be dedicated to helping you.

That is a lot of remote appointments over some time. I am not saying it can't be done, it could. But again, you will need a dedicated professional to do it. Having had that conversation, let's talk about what you need to know about buying hearing aids.

Buying a Hearing Aid

Purchasing a hearing device is a big decision on many levels; firstly, there is a significant financial outlay involved. On top of that is the psychology that seems to be inherent in the decision.

It never fails to surprise me, the deep thoughts and stigma around hearing aids, but you aren't old, it isn't a sign of you losing it, it merely is. Let's take a look at the psychology of it.

The Price is Important, But so are Other Factors

Many first time buyers focus on the price of the instruments; I can understand that because they tend to be expensive. There are many other factors that you need to consider when you are thinking about buying hearing aids.

But let's focus on the price for a minute; generally, the price of a hearing aid includes a lot of services, in fact, years of it. For years I have spoken about unbundling prices, so it is clearer what you are paying for, not many have done it. I believe that will probably change though as pressure to justify cost increases.

I base the price I charge for hearing aids on a simple calculation:

Hearing aid cost + (How much my time is worth x how much time I spend with you) = Hearing Aid Price

I will go into the price considerations in a more in-depth manner later, but here I want to give a quick overview and talk about White Label hearing aids.

Hearing aid price breakdown

If you want to understand what you are paying for, an understanding of the price structure is essential. Generally and certainly in the UK and Ireland, you are paying for the hearing instrument itself and all of the care and support that you is delivered for the lifetime of the device.

All of the private hearing aid dispensers in the UK and Ireland offer a similar service. Professionals in the US generally provide precisely the same thing. It would help if you were clear on what is on offer to you, however.

Because with that knowledge, you can make an educated decision. The general Patient Journey that is on offer is as follows:

The fitting of the hearing aid

The first fitting appointment is then followed by fine-tuning visits to ensure that we customise the hearing aid for you (perhaps two or three visits). The last appointment in this cycle should also involve Real Ear Measurements.

These are crucial visits, and we set the whole foundation of your success with hearing aids during this time. After that, you will be offered either six-monthly or yearly follow up appointments to service the hearing devices and ensure you are still doing fine.

During these visits you can expect to have your ears checked, the hearing aids checked and at least once a year your hearing checked.

The lifetime of a Hearing Aid

You may hear it said that the lifetime of a hearing aid is four to five years, that's not entirely true. Generally when people talk like that, what they mean is that the lifetime of hearing aid technology is four to five years.

By that, I mean that innovation in the hearing aid world tends to move in four-year cycles. Every four to five years, something new comes out that is truly extraordinary in comparison to what went before.

The lifetime of a hearing aid, however, can be up to about ten years, after eight it can become challenging to get it repaired if it fails. So during that period, you are going to attend a lot of half-hour to hour-long appointments with your hearing professional.

That is what you are paying for, time and professional expertise. When you have paid for it, please don't be embarrassed about taking it up. I think that my time is worth money, just like any other professional who offers service when you have paid me for that time; I always make sure that you get it.

Going For the Cheapest Price?

There can be a disparity in prices across different providers, and it can be attractive to go for the cheapest option. What you have to ask yourself is, "is it like for like?" That is the most critical question that you need to ask yourself; later, in the hearing aid section, I discuss hearing aids and their technology levels. I do that so that you can consider this question in a more educated manner.

The lowest price is not always the best option; you need to know all the facts surrounding that price and the equipment and service offered before you can make an educated decision.

What service will they provide, what exactly are the hearing aids, are they the latest technology? Will the professional use Real Ear Measurements to verify or validate that the hearing aids are working as they should? When you have answers to these questions, it is easier to make decisions.

White Label Hearing Aids

Some corporate providers offer white label hearing aids; white-label hearing aids are devices made by manufacturers with a unique label. For instance, Specsavers has the Advance range.

Hidden Hearing has their range which is made by Oticon, in the US Costco has the Kirkland range which was created by Resound, was then made by Signia and is now made by Phonak. Starkey has a white label for its retailers.

I'm not too fond of white label ranges, I understand the commercial reason behind them, but it makes them hard to analyse for the consumer. That is **precisely** why they use a white label, to make it difficult to do like for like comparison.

It is easy for a Dispenser to say oh they are the same as such and such, more often than not, they aren't. The same manufacturer may have made them, but how are you to know what they are exactly?

The information is never really forthcoming, maybe it is my natural sense of suspicion, but why do they need to hide the brand name in the first place?

There is much information to take in when you are buying a hearing aid, and it is easy to feel overwhelmed by the sheer amount of information that you need to consider. That information is both medical and technical.

Medical when it comes to your hearing loss and technical when you are trying to understand any hearing aid technology recommendations.

There is a considerable choice in both types of hearing aid available, and the manufacturers who make them. It can be quite difficult for a consumer to understand it all and sort through what is essential.

A good hearing care professional will help you on that journey, deciphering the gobbledygook. Before we move onto hearing aids and their technology, I want to take a look at the experience of buying a hearing aid, what should happen, and why.

The Hearing Test

The quality and comprehensiveness of the hearing test are essential. It would help if you got a complete hearing test undertaken by a qualified professional. We build our understanding of your ability to hear through many different criteria.

The benefit delivered of varying test procedures like speech audiometry and speech in noise testing to the eventual fit of a hearing aid was once debatable.

However, with recent changes in hearing aids and our increased understanding of hearing loss, the more in-depth the test is, the better the recommendation of a hearing aid and eventual fit.

Information derived from speech testing and speech in noise testing, in particular, is valuable in understanding which hearing aid is best for you.

Speech testing helps us understand how you process speech and what your speech discrimination score may be. QuickSIN or quick Speech In Noise testing tells us a lot about how you process speech in noise.

That is critical information when it comes to choosing a hearing solution, and I say a solution for a good reason. During the QuickSIN test, we will present you with six sentences in increasing levels of background noise.

You simply have to repeat the sentence. We are particularly interested in how you hear five particular words in each sentence. We score you on how many you get in each sentence.

Many of us will present you with two lists, even with the two lists, the test takes no more than five minutes.

We score the test on a 0 to 25 scale based on your ability to repeat the sentences. The scores fall within four bands which are:

- 0 to 3dB: May hear better than normal hearing people in noise with hearing aids

- 3 to 7dB: May hear almost as well as normal hearing people in noise with hearing aids

- 7 to 15dB: Directional mics help, consider an array mic (start to consider accessories)

- Greater than 15dB: Maximum Signal to Noise Ratio improvement needed. Consider FM system

The test allows us to understand your ability to process speech in noise, and it also gives us a clear indication of what you need to get a chance to understand speech in noisy situations.

That matters, because it allows us to give you better recommendations on hearing solutions that will help you and what you can expect from them.

The score is essential for best recommendation, for instance, if you score below 7, well then many modern mid-level technology hearing aids are going to make a massive difference to your ability to hear in noise.

If you score between 7 and 15, well then higher-level technology hearing aids will give you the best opportunity to hear in noise or mid-level hearing aids with wireless accessories.

If you score over 15, well then you need to consider good hearing aids and probably wireless accessories such as remote microphones or FM accessories such as the Roger Pen or Roger Select from Phonak.

That is the only way you will get an opportunity to hear speech in noise well. The test also allows me to set your expectations, recommendations are recommendations, but budget is budget.

If I can help you clearly understand what the hearing aids that you can afford can do for you, that is both good for you and me.

You clearly understand the expectations that can be reasonably be delivered by your aids. I am honest and clear about what the solution can provide. That's good for everyone.

Ideally, we should do most audiological tests in a soundproof booth for complete accuracy, or at a stretch a quiet room. Although with the advent of new types of audiometers designed to eliminate outside noise that is beginning to change.

The consultation should also incorporate more than just testing procedures. To understand your hearing needs, a hearing health professional should discuss your medical history, lifestyle needs and the issues you are having.

Let's go off in a tangent for a minute (as my long-suffering wife says I infuriatingly do often), for me, a significant part of understanding your lifestyle needs is a document called the COSI (Client Orientated Scale of Improvement).

The COSI and Why it is Important

Understanding your hearing loss and its impact on your life is very important for both you and the professional. It is only through the complete understanding that you can then assess how well you are doing if you decide to get hearing aids.

The COSI (Client Orientated Scale of Improvement) is a simple but powerful document designed by the National Acoustic Laboratory, an Australian hearing research body.

You use the document to identify the areas you are having problems in, detail the impact, score how you are doing now, and then come back to it later to score it again after treatment.

But it is much more potent than just a tickbox exercise when appropriately used, let me explain.

The Problems

The COSI should be undertaken during your initial hearing assessment, although, in fairness, it can be conducted anytime during the process.

NAL designed the form to identify the problem areas you are experiencing and grade the difficulties you are experiencing. Key to the power of the document is your commitment to exploring the challenges and being honest about them and the impact they have.

Give Details

A Good COSI thoroughly details the situation, so a simple, when I am talking in groups won't suffice. Detail the situation that you are considering. So something like, I like to meet up with a group of people once a week, once the conversation is in full flow, I have real problems understanding everyone around the table.

Or, my Grandson comes to visit once a week, and when he talks to me, he speaks very softly, I find it very difficult to understand what he is saying.

Or my partner and I watch the TV together every evening. We like to watch a particular show, and the level of volume needs to be much higher for me, which they find a bit too loud.

Talk About The Impact

More than just giving a detailed description, talk about the impact of the problem on you, be honest. No bullshit, big girl and big boy pants on honest.

If you are frustrated by the problem, say it, if you are worried that the problem is affecting your relationships, say it. If it makes you feel lost or lonely, say it. Detail the emotional impact on you from these problems.

No Bullshit Big Girl or Big Boy Pants Honest

Being honest about the impact of hearing loss allows you to acknowledge the emotions involved. It is one of the first steps to understanding what is going on and addressing it. It will also enable you to outline where you are and hopefully motivate you to deal with it.

One of the first steps to getting over the emotional impact of something is acknowledging it so that you can move on.

You will not be the first person to say that you feel you are losing who you are. You will not be the first person to say that you are hugely frustrated; you will not be the first person to say that you feel grief over a loss.

You will not be the first person to say that you feel it is better not to interact rather than be embarrassed. These are natural reactions, don't be embarrassed by them, don't be unwilling to discuss them.

Score Them

When you have finished detailing the problems and the real impact, score how you feel you are doing in those situations. You have finished laying the foundation once you have done that, you have set the true terms of your problems, and you now can assess your ongoing journey with it.

Measuring Your Outcomes

Revisit the COSI on an ongoing basis during your hearing aid journey, score each situation as it is with your hearing aids. During your initial rehab period, you will see your score improve exponentially. At the end of the initial rehab and fine-tuning period, you can look at a final score for your improvement in each situation.

It isn't finished there though, during your long term journey with your hearing aids, you can re-visit the COSI many times. It will tell you where you started in your journey and what your ongoing outcomes have been. You can also use it to identify new situations as your journey progresses and your lifestyle changes.

The COSI is all about you, and it will help you to put everything into perspective, identify and acknowledge the emotional impact and finally allow you to assess your progress. That's not bad for a simple piece of paper.

You can download the COSI for free at: COSI and HAUQ, https://www.nal.gov.au/products/downloadable-software/cosi-and-hauq/

Okay, rant done, let's get back to the test. After the professional completes the test, they should explain to you the severity of your hearing loss and what type of hearing loss it is.

They should also be able to discuss your ability to understand speech in noise. At this point, they should be able to recommend to you which kind of hearing aids and which technology level will work best for you, your lifestyle needs and your hearing loss.

Let's take a more granular look at the hearing test and the different processes.

The hearing test appointment will usually last between one and one and one-half hour. The test includes several different parts that allow a professional to understand the full background to any hearing loss, any medical issues about your hearing and your ability to hear.

Each part of the process offers different information that helps to make recommendations. Each piece of the process has a specific value and will shape the recommendations made. After the hearing test is complete, the professional will explain what they have found and will make recommendations on those findings.

What happens during the hearing test?

Generally, the hearing test, no matter where you get it, will follow the same pattern with similar components. Components within the overall may differ based on who is providing the analysis and the results they are getting.

For instance, some professionals may not undertake speech in noise tests at all; they really should because they offer a lot of value. They may not conduct middle ear testing unless it is required. The hearing test will usually include:

- Examination of the ear and auditory canal, including video otoscopy (camera shows you your ear canal)
- Case history
- A good lifestyle questionnaire
- A full audiometric hearing assessment that will consist of pure tone testing, middle ear testing and speech testing in quiet and noise.
- Explanation and discussion of the outcome
- Impartial advice on the most suited hearing system for your requirements

Let's talk about those stages in more depth.

Otoscopy (Examination of the ear)

This part of the assessment is about the health of your ear, your outer ear and your ear canal. The professional will first examine the outside of your ear using a light.

They are looking for any blemishes strange marks or sore spots. They will then use an instrument called an otoscope to examine your ear canal and your tympanic membrane (eardrum).

They will check the appearance and something called the light response on the eardrum; this is simply the way the light reflects on the drum. A healthy tympanic membrane (eardrum) will reflect the light in a specific way.

This examination may also give indications of problems with your middle ear and signs of any history of perforations. It also allows a professional to become a little familiar with your ear canal. Each ear canal is different, different sizes, different bends.

Many professionals will often use a camera (video otoscopy) to record images of your ear canal and eardrum. Yayyy, you get to see inside your head, or at least your ear canal. Once the professional is happy, they will move onto the next part.

Case History

We take a case history to get an understanding of the background of your hearing loss. During the case history, we will ask typical questions such as your name, address and date of birth.

They will ask you about any treatments in the past that may have used ototoxic drugs (medicines that are toxic to the structures of the inner ear).

Then the professional will ask you questions about any background to the hearing loss. They will try to understand your working history when you noted an issue and if the problem occurred suddenly, has it worsened suddenly, do you have tinnitus, if so is it in only one ear.

These last few questions allow the professional to assess if there is a referrable condition. If they find this to be so, they may well continue the test but will refer you on for further examination by an ENT professional.

Once finished, the professional will also ask you questions about the perception that you have of the impact of your problem on your daily life.

These questions are essential because they allow the professional to begin to understand your lifestyle and the impact if any that hearing loss is having on it.

Sometimes these questions may seem odd, but to get a good understanding of what is best for you, we need to have a good idea of who you are and what you enjoy doing. This is where the previously mentioned COSI comes in.

Some professionals will use it, and others won't. I use it all the time to the best of my ability. Some people aren't as forthcoming as others, but that's okay. It still gives me an idea of the important lifestyle issues.

After they finish the case history, they will move onto the auditory testing proper.

Auditory Testing

Auditory testing is made up of several tests that assess the full function of your hearing system. The examination must be comprehensive, but certain parts of the test may not be needed depending on results from earlier tests.

What happens during auditory testing?

As we said, the professional may not undertake all of the tests discussed here, for instance, you may not need masking and middle ear analysis; however, best practice auditory testing involves the following criteria;

- Pure tone testing (audiometry)
- Masking (audiometry)
- Speech in quiet testing
- Speech in noise testing
- Tympanometry
- Acoustic Reflex Threshold testing
- Distortion Product Otoacoustic Emissions (DPOAE) testing

Audiometry (Hearing Test)

Audiometry or pure tone testing is a series of tests where pure tones (sound like whistles and chirps) or warble tones (similar but they oscillate or vary) are presented through a set of headphones, insert earphones or a bone conduction headband.

57

The professional must undertake both air conduction (through headphones) and bone conduction (through bone conduction headband) tests.

Air conduction audiometry tells us what you can hear from the outside in; bone conduction audiometry tells us what your best inner ear can hear in isolation. The testing is necessary because sometimes there can be a difference and this is the most precise method to identify if you have either sensorineural, conductive or indeed a mixture of both hearing losses.

The professional plots the test results on an audiogram, which shows your hearing sensitivity in the tested frequencies. These tests tell us the softest sound that you can hear and allows us to tell you if your hearing sensitivity is within the normal range or if there is a hearing loss.

Audiometry results tell us many things beyond just your hearing sensitivity; it allows us to see if there is an asymmetry in your hearing loss (a hearing sensitivity that is not equal between the two ears).

It also allows us to see the configuration of your hearing loss (the shape of the way your hearing loss occurs tell us a lot about your hearing loss causes). The test combined with other procedures can help towards a diagnosis of ear abnormalities.

How is audiometry performed?

The initial test involves you carefully listening through headphones (air conduction) that are placed over the ears or insert earphones placed in the ear canals. Pure tones will be presented with the headphones or insert earphones. This part of the test is called air conduction testing and allows the professional to assess what you can hear from the outer ear.

If you hear the sound, you will push a button or raise your hand in response. The professional will continuously reduce the volume of the sound until you can no longer hear it. The key here is that the professional is trying to identify the softest sound you can hear.

So no matter how soft it is if you think you hear it, you should push the button. Many people are never sure and feel like they are letting down the professional.

That couldn't be further than the truth, just relax and don't get frustrated. Once the hearing care professional has finished the headphone or earphone test, the professional will then change to a bone conduction vibrator on a headband. The vibrator is placed behind the ear or sometimes in the middle of your forehead.

This part of the test helps us to find out what your inner ear can hear, it is very rarely different, but in cases of conductive hearing loss, there will be a marked difference.

This part of the test is essential; a previously unidentified conductive hearing loss is a referrable condition. Even if you know that you have a conductive hearing loss and an ENT has assessed it, the results are still crucial for the recommendation and programming of any hearing aids.

This overall test will determine your hearing thresholds and would typically be the end of the audiometry testing. However, just occasionally, the results will point us to undertake advanced audiometry. That is where we earn our money!

Additional tests called masking may be added to the group of tests if we find an asymmetry of thresholds or if you have a conductive hearing loss. Masking is essential, and there are clear rules when a professional needs to do it.

Masking keeps one ear busy while we test the other. In essence, we only do it when we do not trust our initial results.

As I said, there are clear rules on when we should mask and when we should not trust results. You will know masking because the professional will play a white noise type sound in one ear which they will tell you to ignore while they ask you to respond to the regular beeps or whistles in the other.

Speech Testing

We present words at a comfortable listening level, using either free field (through a calibrated speaker) or headphones. You will have to repeat the words, and the professional will score you on the results.

This test gives the professional a deeper understanding of how you hear speech; it also identifies the speech sounds you are missing. After the speech in quiet, the professional will start the QuickSIN (Quick Speech In Noise) test, which I discussed earlier.

I do believe that this test is an essential part of the assessment; it gives the professional a lot of information about how you perceive speech and the signal to noise ratio you need to hear and understand speech in noise.

Why is it important?

The level of sound you hear is only a starting point for our understanding of the impact of your hearing loss. It tells us your ability to hear a sound. Speech testing allows us to understand how well the brain centres that manage hearing are working.

It is often the case that speech scores can be radically different between two people, even if the audiogram results are the same. The speech in noise testing also allows us to understand what type of hearing aid technology level is most suitable for your hearing loss.

For the best diagnosis and hearing aid recommendation, the QuickSIN testing protocol has become a must. It isn't that these tests have a direct impact on the programming of a hearing aid in the same way that the audiogram does.

However, they provide a deeper understanding of your speech understanding problems and allow us to explain them, and why we are recommending a particular hearing aid or hearing aid technology.

How is speech testing performed?

Most independent hearing health professionals have updated their testing equipment to allow them to run automated speech and speech in noise tests through their audiometer. During these tests, they will ask you to repeat words that are presented to you at normal speech volume levels with and without noise.

Word recognition scores will be determined and recorded on their system. The QuickSIN test will give a signal to noise ratio score, which will provide a professional with a clear idea about the hearing devices that will help you in noise. It will also give a clear indication that you might need assistive devices to get the best possible opportunity to hear. I will address that a little later in the section called "What if hearing aids aren't enough?"

Middle Ear Analysis

What is middle ear analysis?
We undertake middle ear analysis tests to assess the function of the middle ear. The tests will determine how sound travels through your middle ear and also how your brain reacts to some sounds. You will feel a shortlived blocked sensation while a recording takes place.

These tests are not necessarily that important in the usual run of the mill hearing loss; they only become relevant if there is a clear need for them. So if I have identified that there is a mid-ear issue, Tympanometry will help me understand what that issue might be.

Tympanometry itself will not have any bearing on either the hearing aid that is fitted or the programming of that hearing aid; the audiometric results will. There are two parts to the Middle Ear Assessment: Tympanometry and Acoustic Reflexes.

Tympanometry

What is tympanometry?
It consists of measuring how much your eardrums are moving and if that movement is within normal limits. It tells us if there is any fluid or congestion behind the eardrums. (Presence of fluid

behind one's eardrums is known as glue ear, and it is prevalent in children).

This test measures how well your middle ear works. Your middle ear includes your eardrum, the middle ear bones, and your Eustachian tube. It will reveal abnormalities which will signify and can explain a conductive hearing loss and/or a sensation of pressure in the ear.

How is tympanometry performed?

We place an ear tip in the canal connected to a handheld machine; it briefly varies the pressure in the ear while playing a tone. By changing the pressure, we can measure the movement of the eardrum. It takes only a few minutes to complete. You will not need to respond to this test.

Acoustic Reflex Thresholds

What is acoustic reflex threshold testing?

When we hear a loud noise, our ear protects itself with a reflex which stiffens the eardrum. We use this reflex to test the Facial and Auditory nerves. This test measures how the stapedius muscle contracts in response to a loud sound. The absence or presence of acoustic reflexes can be necessary for differential diagnosis.

How is acoustic reflex threshold testing performed?

Often, we undertake tympanometry and acoustic reflex thresholds together. With the ear tip in your canal, you will hear progressively louder beeps. You will not need to respond. Instead, the machine will automatically measure the response.

Distortion Product Oto-acoustic Emissions (DPOAE)

What is DPOAE testing?

This test measures how well the outer hair cells in the cochlear work. The outer hair cells produce low-level sounds called Otoacoustic Emissions in response to clicks. A conductive or sensorineural hearing loss will often result in absent DPOAE responses.

How is DPOAE testing performed?

With an ear tip in the canal, clicks are presented in the ear. In response, the cochlear emits a sound which is recorded by the equipment. The extent of the response and the frequency at which the response occurs is measured and recorded.

Explanation of the results

Once the testing is complete, the professional will explain the results, they will explain what they have found and detail why it is having the impact it is in your life. They will also make recommendations based on their results for you to return to a more normal level of hearing and allow you to engage fully in your life.

Hearing Aid Benefit Assessment

If you are a suitable candidate for hearing aids, many professionals will then move onto a hearing aid benefit assessment or demonstration.

In essence, what they will do is programme a set of demo hearing aids to your loss, they will not give you full amplification but a level close to it.

The demo will allow you a taste of what hearing aids sound like and how they will work. Any professional worth their salt will move through a demonstration of different features explaining to you as they go what they are and how they will work for you.

Go to the Test Accompanied

You should always take a loved one with you to your hearing test; firstly, undergoing any medical examination or procedure can be stressful. It is always a good idea to take someone with you to a medical appointment.

While caught up in the process and worrying about results, it is easy to miss other relevant information. If you have someone with you, they can help to remember what was said. Two people retain much more information.

On this point, feel free to make notes during the appointment and don't be nervous about asking questions. Query anything that you do not fully understand. Conversely, don't be afraid to ask the professional to write something down for you.

A true professional will not upset by being asked questions; these questions will come up; it is better to ask them at the appointment. As a professional, we understand that this experience is new to you, and the information is foreign.

We also know that it is our job to help you understand. It is also essential to have your family involved in the process.

Hearing Loss is a Family Sport

Hearing loss affects every member of the family, not just the person who suffers from it. Communication is a problem; often frustrations creep in for everyone. Family members may feel that the person with hearing loss is in denial or just ignoring the impact of the hearing loss.

If the person with hearing loss has withdrawn from their social circle, family members may be concerned about their well-being. Hearing loss tends to affect the entire family.

Denial is Not Just a River in Egypt

A grand old Dublin saying, "De Nile is not just a river in Egypt", usually uttered as someone shakes their head and throws their eyes to heaven. There is much talk about denial in hearing loss, and there is undoubtedly an element of denial involved in many cases. However, the misunderstanding of how hearing loss works feeds that denial.

Cultural Understanding of Hearing Loss

Firstly, most people don't understand how acquired hearing loss works or how it will affect someone's ability to hear. We form our understanding of hearing loss through what we see on TV and hear on Radio and the Theatre stage.

In that world, hearing loss is not just something to laugh at; it appears to be all about raising the volume. "Speak Up, Speak UP, What Did You Say?" It is all very Monty Pythonesque.

Hearing Loss is rarely about Pure Volume

Run of the mill acquired hearing loss is very rarely about volume; it is nearly always about balance in sound. Hearing loss that is about pure brute force volume is quite rare, and it is usually something present from, or related to, something from birth.

In average, run of the mill acquired hearing loss, there is an imbalance in the ability to hear sounds. You can hear some sounds quite well, while you may not be able to hear other sounds at all.

I Can Hear The Voice!

Quite often, someone with hearing loss can hear someone's voice very clearly; they can't understand what some of the words are. If you think about that for a minute, you can see why it is easy to believe that the problem is, in fact, the speaker, not the listener.

If they can hear the voice, surely the problem is that the speaker isn't speaking clearly enough? The actual problem is that more often than not, someone with hearing loss can't hear consonants in speech.

So basically words sound indistinct and mumbled. The person isn't mumbling; you just can't hear them properly. However, you can see why it is easy to think that the problem is the speaker rather than your own.

That is why people take so long to realise they are having problems. It is also why they are reluctant to release the idea that it isn't them, it's everyone else.

Helping You Make a Realisation

When family members attend a hearing test, they will often help their loved one towards a realisation about their hearing ability. It is the family who understands the effect of hearing loss on the person who has it. They see and understand when there are problems, more transparently than the person who is suffering them.

Don't forget, as a person with hearing loss; you don't miss what you have missed. Or to put it another way, you don't know what you don't hear. People around you do. While you may be unsure about the depth of the problems you are having, the people around you tend to see them clearly.

I have often witnessed a Patient come to a clear realisation of their issues solely through the testament of a family member. Quite often, it is the first time that they undertake a discussion about their hearing in a clear and focused manner.

More often than not, it also leads to the sharing of worries that have been unsaid. Concern that has often been unvoiced.

Keeping You Honest

The other thing that a family member will often do is to keep you honest. I have spoken here and on the Hearing Aid Know site about not fooling yourself. As I said, family members tend to see what is happening and generally aren't afraid to give you the unvarnished truth.

Nor are they afraid to speak up when you are lying to yourself. Loved ones have a way of telling you how it is. I find the reaction to hearing loss a bizarre thing; it seems to be one of the few health issues that are surrounded by personal stigma.

Hearing loss is not a statement about you; it just is!

People will outright lie to themselves about their ability to hear to protect themselves from the thoughts in their heads! It never fails to surprise me, I have said it before, and I have no doubt I will repeat it, hearing loss is not a statement about you, it just is.

Helping Them Understand

Your family doesn't understand hearing loss any more than you do. Attending the appointment will also allow them to understand the issues. It will also enable them to become familiar with your hearing loss and the effects it has on your ability to communicate. The hearing test will make it very clear to them precisely what the issues are and why you have the problems you do.

Moving Forward

If you move forward with hearing aids, the involvement of your family with your ongoing rehabilitation plan is essential. They need to understand the advantages and limitations of the hearing aids you have chosen. They also need to know how they can help you, especially during the early stages of rehabilitation.

A Better Understanding of Progress

As you move forward with hearing aids, family members can also help to assess your progress. They can also help identify areas where you are still having issues with your hearing. I love when family members are involved in the process; they are a secondary source of information which allows a full picture of what is going on. They are also a validation of the problems. Let me explain that.

When someone has an issue hearing, they automatically think it is their hearing loss and the fault of the hearing aids. Sometimes, it isn't. There have been times where a Patient has spoken about problems with a particular situation or a specific person.

The family member has chimed in and said, and I hadn't a clue what they were saying either! Or I couldn't make it out with all the noise going on either. In essence, if they can't hear, neither should the Patient be able to.

In contrast to that, some Patients may think they are doing pretty well in some situations and the family member may be able to point out where there are some deficiencies.

The inclusion of the family in the process is a good thing for both the Patient and for them. So get your family involved early.

Understanding Hearing Loss

So the test is finished, and the hearing care professional is explaining your hearing loss while pointing at a fancy graph, using words like low-frequency and high-frequency, sensorineural and bi-lateral. What the hell does that gobbledygook mean? Let's talk about hearing loss, reading an audiogram, the types of damage and the effects.

Many different problems can cause hearing loss, a few of which can be successfully treated with medicine or surgery, depending on the disease process. Unfortunately, we can't treat most forms of hearing loss with anything other than hearing aids. Up to recently, professionals generally discussed three types of hearing loss.

However, in the recent past, a new type of hearing impairment has gained recognition. Auditory processing disorder is not your typical hearing loss; however, the problems caused by the condition fit within the symptoms of typical hearing loss. Let's talk about types of hearing loss.

Conductive Hearing Loss

Diseases or obstructions in the outer or middle ear cause conductive losses that usually affect all frequencies of hearing. Some conductive hearing losses are temporary, and some are chronic or long term. Conductive loss can often be medically treated sometimes with surgery.

We treat Temporary conductive losses (usually caused by mid-ear infections) with medication. For a conductive hearing loss of a more chronic nature, a hearing aid is generally a fantastic solution delivering real benefit.

What can cause a conductive hearing loss?

Anything that interferes with the transmission of sound from the outer to the inner ear will cause a conductive hearing loss. That could be a malformation of the outer ear, ear canal, or middle ear structures, or a perforated eardrum (surgical correction may be possible).

Fluid buildup in the middle ear caused by colds or upper respiratory tract infections will create a temporary hearing loss (temporary, should pass with the condition that caused it).

Ear infection formally called otitis media, (an infection of the middle ear that causes an accumulation of fluid) will interfere with the movement of the eardrum and ossicles (this can be temporary, but chronic ongoing otitis media can cause permanent damage). so the causes of a conductive hearing loss can be classified as:

- Middle ear infections (otitis media).
- Collection of fluid in the middle ear ("glue ear" in children).
- Blockage of the outer ear, most commonly by wax.
- Otosclerosis, a condition in which the ossicles of the middle ear harden and become less mobile.
- Damage to the ossicles, for example by severe infection or head injury.
- Cholesteatoma (growth usually in the attic of the middle ear)
- Perforated (pierced) eardrum, which can be caused by an untreated ear infection, head injury or a blow to the ear, or from poking something in your ear.

Sensorineural Hearing Loss

A sensorineural loss results from some damage to the inner ear (cochlea). Sometimes referred to as a nerve-related hearing loss or nerve deafness. The hearing loss can range from mild to profound and often affects specific frequencies more than others. The only treatment for sensorineural hearing loss at present is hearing aids.

What is the cause of sensorineural hearing loss?

A sensorineural hearing loss is due to damage to the pathway that sound impulses take from the hair cells of the inner ear to the auditory nerve and the brain. So sensorineural hearing loss happens when there is damage to the structures of the inner ear (cochlea), disease, noise or genetic issues can cause it.

It can also be damage to the nerve that runs from the inner ear to the brain (auditory nerve). That can be caused by disease, tumour or genetic issues.

Finally, damage to the auditory centre of the brain, with varying causes such as disease or stroke. Generally speaking, the origins of sensorineural hearing loss tend to be the following:

- Age-related hearing loss (presbyacusis). This is the natural decline in hearing that many people experience as they get older. It's partly due to the loss of hair cells in the cochlea.
- Acoustic trauma (injury caused by loud noise) can damage hair cells.
- Certain viral or bacterial infections such as mumps or meningitis can lead to loss of hair cells or other damage to the auditory nerve.
- Ménière's disease, which causes dizziness, tinnitus, and hearing loss.
- Certain drugs, such as some powerful antibiotics, can cause permanent hearing loss. At high doses, we believe that aspirin can cause temporary tinnitus – a persistent ringing in the ears. The antimalarial drug quinine can also cause tinnitus, but it's not thought to cause permanent damage.

- Acoustic neuroma. This is a benign (non-cancerous) tumour affecting the auditory nerve. It needs to be observed and will be treated with surgery.
- Other neurological (affecting the brain or nervous system) conditions such as multiple sclerosis, stroke, or a brain tumour.

Mixed Hearing Loss

A mixed loss is as it sounds a mix of both conductive and sensorineural hearing losses that occur in both the inner and outer or middle ear. A mixed hearing loss tends to be pretty rare.

What are the causes of Mixed Hearing Loss?

A combination of conductive damage in the outer or middle ear and sensorineural damage in the inner ear (cochlea) or nerve of hearing causes mixed hearing loss.

The causes for both are the same as they are in isolation, so for the conductive loss, it can be middle ear issues, eardrum issues or even an outer ear problem. For the sensorineural problem, it can be genetics, noise exposure or disease.

Auditory Processing Disorder

Auditory Processing Disorder or APD is a catch-all term for hearing difficulties caused by central processing disorders. In most cases, a person may have a completely normal audiogram, but their ability to understand speech in noise is compromised. For this reason, the broader media have dubbed it Hidden Hearing Loss.

What Causes APD?

We don't know; there have been many theories, such as acquired injury to the processing centres of the brain at birth. It may also be genetic issues that cause processing problems or developmental in that something may occur that compromises hearing during an especially important time of development in the auditory processing area of the brain.

For instance, there has been considerable interest in chronic otitis media in children and its effect on auditory processing during an especially important time of learning and speech development.

The Audiogram

The audiogram is the name of the graph that professionals use to plot your hearing test results. You can see an image below which I have taken from our audiogram tool on Hearing Aid Know.

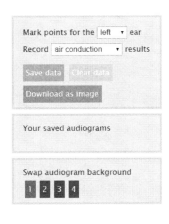
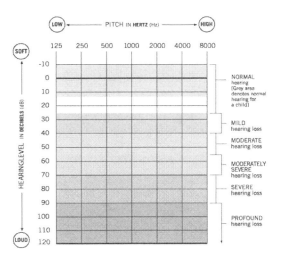

Frequencies or Pitch

On the top of the audiogram, you will see the pitch in Hertz marked with the numbers 125, 250, 500 etc. These represent different sound frequencies. They represent the sound frequencies that are most important for speech.

The 1000 Hz line is the midpoint with everything below it being low-frequency and everything above it being high frequency. That's not exactly true, but it will do for this explanation.

What Does it Mean For Speech

Low-frequency sounds in speech are the vowel sounds in words. They are the power of speech. High-frequency sounds are the consonant sounds in speech. The consonant sounds in speech help form the words; they give them the context needed to be understood.

A person with a general run of the mill hearing loss often has difficulty in understanding words or parts of words. That is because their high-frequency hearing is usually worse than their low-frequency hearing. As I said earlier, they can hear the voice well enough; they just aren't sure what you are saying.

When speaking, the voice may be audible, but separate words may sound mixed up or blurred together. Rhyming words, or terms that are similar such as cat/cap, bread/thread, pool/cool, etc. are challenging to distinguish when the listener has a hearing loss.

More often than not, this is because the person with hearing loss does not hear the consonant sounds very well, if at all. The fact that low-frequency hearing is better or normal in some cases compounds the issues caused by high-frequency loss. That is because all background noise is low-frequency. The ability to hear it well helps to mask the high-frequency cues even more.

Volume or Intensity

To the left-hand side of the graph, you see the numbers -10 to 120. These denote the level of intensity or volume of a given sound. The audiogram uses dB HL (dB Hearing Loss). You will note a thick black line across the audiogram at 0, and this line represents normal hearing.

However, everyone's normal is different, and for the purpose of testing hearing, anything between -10 and 25 is normal. In terms of speech, 40 to 45 dB is soft speech, 65 dB is normal conversational speech, and finally, 80 to 85 dB is loud speech.

Severity of Loss

To the right-hand side of the audiogram, you will see areas denoted with the severity of hearing loss. Which run from mild through to profound.

Audiogram Markings

As we test your hearing, we mark the audiogram with the lowest level of sound you can hear, frequency, by frequency and ear by ear. When we finish, the audiogram shows us the shape of your hearing loss and the severity.

The markings used are generally, red Os for the right ear for air conduction results (through the headphones). Blue Xs for the left ear for air conduction results. Green triangles for bone conduction results. If we have undertaken masking, black symbols such as these], [will be seen.

If the bone conduction results are close to or on top of the air conduction results. Then the hearing loss is sensorineural (inner ear damage). If the bone conduction results are better than the air conduction results, well then there is some sort of conductive hearing loss (middle ear issue).

Hearing Loss Descriptions

We use descriptions for hearing loss based on the shape of the audiogram, the severity of the loss and the type of hearing loss. For instance, we would use descriptions such as sloping mild to moderate sensorineural hearing loss, or moderate high-frequency or flat severe hearing conductive hearing loss. We use those terms both to quantify the loss and help you to understand the results.

The Hearing Aids

If the professional recommends a set of hearing instruments, don't be afraid to ask them to write the details down for you if you wish to research them. As I said, some companies may offer white label instruments.

These instruments are re-named by the manufacturers, specifically for the company. If they offer a white label, ask who is the manufacturer of the device and on what aid it is based.

Don't be nervous about asking questions; ask about the different kinds of hearing aid available which are suitable for your type of hearing loss. Ask why they are recommending those particular hearing aids. As I said, a professional will not be put off by any questions. Don't be afraid to say that you would like to research the hearing aids that they have recommended to you.

On Hearing Aid Know, we try to offer a decent high-level view of most hearing aids to give a good understanding of what they will do for you. My friend Abram Bailey runs a website called Hearing Tracker, you can find it at

www.hearingtracker.com

The site offers rundowns of both hearing providers and hearing aids in the US; it also has consumer reviews of both. It is an excellent place to research the effectiveness of both the hearing aids and the providers who are listed.

Personally speaking, we think that Hearing Aid Know and Hearing Tracker are the very best consumer advice websites for hearing aids. Because they are both independent, tell it like it is websites. Of course, ours is the best one, hahaha.

Hearing Aids, Have Realistic Expectations

You need to have realistic expectations of the hearing aid technology you buy and what it can deliver for you. Modern hearing aids are exceptional pieces of technology, but they are not, nor probably will never be, a replacement for normal hearing.

The higher the technology level of the hearing aid, the better the results for you. Keep this clearly in mind when you are making any purchase decision. Don't buy low technology hearing aids and expect them to help you in all situations; they simply won't.

Knowing What You Want Helps

Before you decide what to buy, have a clear idea of what you want from your hearing aids. Think carefully about your problem situations, consider where solving those problems is essential for you. If you keep that clear, you can consider what type of technology level will be best for you.

If you have a sedentary lifestyle and all you want hearing aids for, is listening to TV and Radio, some light conversation and the occasional journey to the shop. Low-end technology should almost certainly meet all your needs.

However, if you have a busier lifestyle and your hearing aids will be imperative for more complex sound situations, then higher levels of technology are most certainly for you. Key to any decision is the understanding of your needs and realistic expectations of the technology level of hearing aids that you will buy.

With this in mind, you will know what you can expect from what you can afford. When this is clear to you, it will make your journey with your hearing aids less stressful for you. It is the Dispenser's job to make this clear to you and they often will, however, you need to listen.

It isn't a sales technique, they aren't trying to up-sell you, and more often than not, they are merely giving the best advice possible. It is up to you to decide what you get within your budget, just be clear about what that will deliver to you.

Wireless Accessories

In recent years most hearing aid manufacturers have moved towards wireless communication within their hearing aids. This connectivity has opened up new options and resulted in new accessory devices that deliver real benefits for hearing aid users.

You can now purchase many additional extras with your hearing aids. These are all useful add-ons which can help someone with hearing loss to lead the life that they are would like and expect.

I think that these devices are outstanding; however, as with many things; they are only useful if you are going to use them. Each manufacturer will offer some wireless solution, and the question is, do you need them?

These can increase the costs, so think carefully before buying. Don't pay for something which you might not use very often or pay for something you don't need.

However, having said that, if your budget constrains you, and you can't go for the technology level of hearing aids you would like. An accessory can help to make up for what you are missing.

For instance, a wireless remote microphone can deliver fantastic results for hearing in noise even when paired with a low technology hearing aid. Keep this in mind when you are making the buying decision.

Be Sure Of What Are You Buying

So you have decided to buy, you have picked out the aids and the accessory you want. You need to be sure about what you are buying. Ask the seller to explain in detail what you are precisely paying for if they say lifetime aftercare, ask what does that mean?

The life of the hearing aid, a set period, your lifetime? What does that aftercare include, are there structured callbacks, will you drop back when you have a problem, or will they just call you for a re-test in five years?

These are all things that you need to know, I have said it before, hearing aids are sophisticated devices that need care and attention to deliver to their best ability. Hearing problems are not like vision problems, hearing aids are not like glasses, you don't put them on, and everything will be fine.

You need support and rehabilitation, and that support needs to be ongoing. So it is crucial that you clearly understand what you are buying when you pay your money. What aftercare and help will you get?

General Considerations

When choosing the size and shape of an aid, an important consideration is your dexterity. You may find that smaller hearing aids are difficult for you to handle and insert. Not just that, the battery that powers it, maybe too small for you to handle, if your eyesight is not great, you may also have issues with the size of the aid or the battery.

Always remember, you are a customer as well as a Patient, and if you feel that you want to try something different or go away and think about it, then do so. I have mentioned aftercare already, but you must understand what you are buying.

Find out about aftercare and warranty servicing of your hearing aids. They are an expensive investment, and you should always check exactly what they include in the warranty and aftercare service.

Make Sure You Have a Written Agreement

Finally, make sure you have a written agreement, then you always have a reference to the agreement you have made. I sincerely hope that this advice will allow you to make educated hearing healthcare decisions.

Find a company that you feel comfortable with, ask them lots of questions about the hearing aids that they offer, what they think would be best for you and what exactly is their service offering and you should never go wrong.

Better Hearing, an organisation in the States, offers an excellent rundown on buying hearing aids. You can find it here:

http://www.betterhearing.org/hearingpedia/hearing-aids/guide-buying-hearing-aids

What If Hearing Aids Are Not Enough?

Unfortunately, for some people hearing aids will never be enough to help them understand in every situation. No matter what level of hearing aid technology they buy, they will still have problems, sometimes even in moderately noisy situations.

To understand this issue, we need first to discuss speech discrimination, and why people may have these problems. We can then explore strategies that may help.

Why Would Hearing Aids Not Help?

There are two reasons why a set of hearing aids might not help you in certain situations. The first reason is that the level of technology you have bought was never designed to help you in that noisy environment.

The second reason is deeper than the tech, and it involves what is going on in your mechanism of hearing and possibly your auditory cortex. Unfortunately, sometimes no matter what we do with the technology, your ability to understand speech in noisy situations may still be problematic.

Hearing aid technology has moved on so much that it is easy for us as professionals to lose sight of the fact that for some people, they won't work everywhere. I mean, I get excited about hearing aid technology as it evolves, and I see the treatment benefits that the evolution of technology brings.

However, I need to remember that the revolution in hearing aid technology delivers significant benefits to most of the people who need it, not all. In a general run of the mill hearing loss, a good set of hearing aids will work exceptionally well. Depending on the level of technology purchased, they will work well almost everywhere.

However, if you have a hearing loss, which is further compounded by a speech discrimination issue, well then even the most exceptional hearing aids may not be enough for you. Let's talk about speech discrimination and why it matters to the outcomes that you will experience with hearing aids.

Speech Discrimination Score

We measure your ability to hear sounds, and that allows us to understand your hearing loss and the softest sound that you can hear. However, it doesn't give us an indication of your ability to understand or process speech.

To assess your speech discrimination, we measure how well you can understand what you hear when speech is loud enough to hear comfortably.

We measure speech discrimination in per cent terms, so if your discrimination scores are 100%, you understand every word that you hear. However, if your speech discrimination is 0%, you can't understand a single word no matter how loud it is.

It isn't very often that we see 0% scores from anybody with a regular, general run of the mill loss. While hearing loss is a function of damage to your hearing mechanism (outer ear, middle ear and inner ear). Speech discrimination difficulties may not be. We believe that speech discrimination issues can be caused by damage to the outer and inner hair cells in the inner ear. However, there may be central auditory issues at play as well. In essence, the brain may not be sorting out the information as it should.

Generally, speech discrimination problems and hearing loss go hand in hand. However, even somebody with a severe hearing loss may have speech discrimination of 70 or 80%. Which at its basic level means that they understand four out of every five words if presented at the right volume.

Hearing loss levels are not a good indication of speech discrimination. Two people may have the same hearing loss (unlikely but you know an example right) but have two completely different speech discrimination scores. The key to me blathering on here is this if you have a hearing loss and your discrimination is good (80% or higher), typically you will find hearing aids will work pretty damn well for you in most sound environments.

However, if your discrimination is poor, well then hearing aids will not deliver everything that you need to hear better in complex situations (noisy ones). The more complex the situation, the more difficulty you will have. While wearing the top of the range hearing aids will give you a little boost, they will still not deliver everything that you need. So what is the answer to an infuriating problem?

Assistive Listening Devices

If your ability to discriminate speech dives in noisier situations, even when wearing a set of hearing aids, well then you need strategies to help give you an edge. While there are coping mechanisms that may help. The one thing that should dramatically improve things, or at least provide enough help for you to work out what is going on is some sort of assistive listening device.

Every hearing aid brand now offers a range of assistive listening products. Some are specific to one situation or need, while some of the latest ones are multi-functional offering different functionalities in one device. I want to just focus on one device right now because I want to give you an example of how a device can change your life for the better.

The Multi Mic

The Multi Mic device from Resound is both a remote microphone (for a partner to wear) and an intelligent desktop microphone (place it on a table, and it helps pick up a group conversation). However, Resound was not happy with just that, and they also included a line in (attach any audio source to the mic with a cable) and a telecoil receiver (connect wirelessly to loop systems). So you can see when I say multi-functional I mean it.

Of course, the Multi Mic only works with Resound hearing aids. If you are in a noisy situation with just one person, they can wear the multi-mic, and you will hear their voice directly in your hearing aids. If you are in a noisy situation and you are with a small group, you can lay the multi-mic down on the table in front of you, and it will help pick up the voices of your companions and stream them directly into your hearing aids.

The device is intelligent, knows it is laying on a table and changes how its microphones work to catch the voices of the group better. In this way, the device helps to deliver the best and cleanest signal to your ears, giving you the optimum opportunity to work out what is being said.

The telecoil addition is inspired, all public buildings in Ireland and the UK have loop systems, nearly all churches have one, most banks, post offices, theatres, concert halls and cinemas. The loop wirelessly transmits relevant audio and the telecoil picks up that transmission and streams it directly to your hearing aids.

Loop systems are becoming much more common in the US through stalwart work of activists and the Hearing Loss Association of America. The inclusion of a telecoil receiver means that you can wear a discreet pair of hearing aids with no in-built telecoil, but still have access to what is an excellent system through the multi-mic.

The line in speaks for itself, you plug your audio from the television or your music player, and it is streamed directly to your hearing aids. The functionality of these types of devices gives you the best chance to hear enough to work out what is going on.

Personal Experience With Connect Clip

I have had some personal experience with remote mics, I first used the Soundclip-A from Bernafon, and it blew me away. I then used the Connect Clip from Oticon and again was impressed with the functionality (in essence, they are the same device).

Recently, I got a hold of a Resound Multi-Mic, and with my limited use of it have been thoroughly impressed. If you have speech discrimination issues that are particularly exacerbated by noise, well then this type of technology should be a given for you.

More recently, I got a hold of a Roger Pen and a Roger Select from Phonak which worked with a set of Marvel hearing aids I was testing. Roger equipment is expensive, but it is incredible. I was utterly in awe of the benefit the devices offered. You can read more about them in the Phonak section of the book.

Aren't Telecoils Obsolete?

Hell No! You Should Always Consider a Telecoil. I read with horror recently that a professional told a prospective patient that hearing loops and hearing aid telecoils were obsolete technology now replaced by Bluetooth. That is not true, while telecoils and loop systems are old technology, both systems are just as relevant today to prospective hearing aid users as ever.

Even with the ever-growing Bluetooth hearing aid market, a telecoil is still a valid feature and will remain so for many years to come. Manufacturers build some modern hearing aids with both Bluetooth and telecoils for a reason. Let's talk about why you should always consider a telecoil in your hearing aids.

A Looping Resurgence

In the UK, Ireland and most countries in Europe, loop systems are everywhere. In every public building including concert halls, churches, theatres, airports, Taxis, shops and government buildings. Mainly because of the EU's insistence on accessibility for everybody (damn EU making it easy for everyone to be included!).

While that isn't the case in the US, loop systems are seeing a huge resurgence over there because of committed campaigners and the Hearing Loss Association of America. More and more loop systems are coming online in the US in public places.

It's straightforward; telecoils allow you to connect easily to loop systems. Loop systems provide direct wireless audio input into your hearing aids. No interference, no background noise, just the signal directly from the input, whether that is the microphone a priest is using, the audio system in a theatre, the microphone the cashier is speaking into at the bank or the music from the concert hall stage.

The system gives you the very best access to the sound you want to hear. So no, telecoils are not obsolete, they may be old, but they work just fine, and there is no sign of a better solution on the horizon. If anything, loop systems are becoming more popular in the US, so you will get to use your telecoil in more places than ever moving forward.

Fitting the Hearing Aids

So we have covered the hearing test and making your decision about buying hearing aids. Let's talk about the initial fit of the hearing aids and the aftercare. Firstly let's look at the actual fitting of your new hearing aid devices, what do you need to consider and what information should they give to you?

The Fitting

The fitting itself is a relatively short exercise; the professional will place the hearing aids on and programme them to your hearing loss. We would undertake some tests concerning how you are hearing and verify that they are delivering against the targets that we set. The initial prescription level we set will often not be the optimum prescription.

That is so that the hearing aids do not overwhelm you. You will need to acclimatise to them, and this will happen over time. However, we would programme the hearing aids to automatically increase the prescription gently to move you towards the optimum over a period of time.

That is called automatic acclimatisation, and it is something that is done slowly, in fact, you will barely notice that the amplification is changing as you wear them.

Getting Comfortable With Your Hearing Aids

We try to ensure that you are entirely comfortable with your hearing aids. When we say comfortable, we don't just mean physically. You need to be comfortable not just wearing your hearing aids but also handling them. You will be wearing your hearing aids every day, all day. Initially, they will feel odd, in particular, if you are a first time user. However, that should settle down very quickly.

We will make sure that you can insert the hearing aids in, or on, your ears by yourself. We will also ensure that you can take them out with ease. It is vital that you can handle your hearing aids with ease and confidence; otherwise, they will not fulfil their purpose as solutions to deliver you a better life.

The Batteries

The need for batteries is diminishing with the advent of rechargeable hearing aids. However, not all styles of hearing aids are rechargeable, so until that time happens, there will be hearing aid batteries around.

We will show you what batteries you need and how to put the batteries into your hearing aid. We must assess that you can manage the batteries by yourself. We will make sure that you can both handle them and put them in.

We will also give you information on where you can buy batteries, how much they cost, and why it is a good idea to keep spare batteries handy. If your hearing aids are rechargeable, we will instruct you on the use of the charger and inserting and taking out the hearing aids from the charger.

Controls on Your Hearing Aids

If your hearing aids have any controls, we will show you how to use them and what they do. You should make sure that you can operate all of the hearing aid controls yourself, and change the listening programmes if there is any. We must assess whether you have the dexterity to operate the controls for your hearing aid. If we supply a remote or accessory with your hearing aid, we will show you how to use it.

Cleaning & Caring For Your Hearing Aids

We will show you how to clean and care for your hearing aid. Hearing aids are a significant investment; taking good care of them makes real financial sense. We will talk about keeping earwax out of the sound bore and changing wax guards if your hearing aid has them. We will also talk about daily cleaning routines and why you should use a dehumidifier box as part of your care routine.

Proper care and maintenance of your hearing aid are crucial, and it will ensure that it continues to help you hear better for longer. At the initial fitting, all of this will just be a quick run-through; we don't want to overload you with information.

We will ask you to read the owner's manual, and at further appointments, we will ensure that we reinforce the information and that you can clean and care for the devices.

Assistive Listening and Alerting Devices

A hearing aid may not be the full answer for you; in some instances, there may be some assistive devices that make sense for you and your lifestyle. Most hearing aid manufacturers have released their own wireless devices for hearing aids.

However, there are many more available from non-hearing aid manufacturers like smoke detectors and amplified phones. We will always give you information regarding assistive listening technology such as the telecoil, mobile phone technology, how best to use phones etc.

Real Ear Measurements

In a conversation with Steve, it became evident that I hadn't taken a real stand on a subject that is important to me. The issue is probe tube measurements of hearing aids. They are more commonly called Real Ear Measurements (REMs) and or Live Speech Mapping.

They are elements of hearing aid verification and validation. They are the best practice, the gold standard in hearing aid fitting. They are a proven strategy for increasing satisfaction with hearing aids and have been for many years.

In fact, as a consumer advice champion, advising you of what they are, what benefit you will derive from them, and why you should demand them is my job.

Let's talk about what they are, how we do them, and why you aren't getting the best service if a hearing care professional doesn't carry them out for you.

Live Speech Mapping and Real Ear Measurements, Why You Need Them During Your Hearing Aid Journey

They are forms of verification of a prescriptive target and validation of a prescriptive target. Let me explain the difference. They designed Real Ear Measurements to verify that the hearing aids in your ears are hitting the objectives prescribed by the fitting prescriptions Nal and DSL.

Those fitting prescriptions have been with us for many years, and the clinical world accepts them as the very best fitting prescriptions. However, not everyone agrees that in the modern world of hearing aids, that Nal or DSL is still the best way forward. Some people, like me, think that hearing aid manufacturers often use their own fitting prescriptions because they know their hearing aids best.

With that in mind, we need a test to see if those non-standard (as such) prescriptions deliver the speech signal required to help people. We can't use REMs to verify because all REM protocols are designed just for Nal and DSL.

However, we can validate it using live speech mapping to ensure that we are amplifying a controlled speech signal into the residual hearing envelope of a Patient.

For me, and it is only a personal opinion, live speech mapping is the better option. That is because I am not necessarily beholden to Nal or DSL.

Why are REMs and Live Speech Mapping Important?

These tests are necessary because they verify or validate that the hearing aid is providing the sound that you need to hear better. The settings take your hearing loss into account and provide the calculations for the amplification required to deliver for you. When we run the tests, we are assessing what is going on in your ear canal.

There is no guessing, no trusting the hearing aids to just work, and it is a clear assessment of whether they are delivering or not. This assessment allows us to make real-time changes to the hearing aid settings to ensure that they do provide the amplification you need.

All of the studies undertaken into the use of verification and validation measures within hearing aid fittings show that people get on better and are more satisfied with their hearing aids when we do REMs.

The Possible Pitfalls

Here is the thing though, when we use these tests, we get the hearing aids to the optimal settings for your hearing loss. You actually might not like the sound, and in fact, you might hate it and need it turned down. I don't see that as a bad thing, neither should you.

The professional will explain to you that you won't get the best possible experience, but we can help you work towards it during your rehabilitation. Just because you might not like the sound, doesn't mean I shouldn't do it, and anyone who uses that excuse is talking rubbish. Utter and contemptuous rubbish.

How is it Done?

We perform both processes in a similar way. We use a probe tube system. The hilarity that ensues when I get to say, "this is where we probe you" followed by a Dr Evil cackle is endless, I told you, my humour, just ignore it.

The system consists of separate devices for each ear that has thin white rubber probes. There is a probe for each ear, and they look like a short straw. First, we calibrate the probe tubes by holding them in front of a speaker, which plays the calibration tones.

We need to do the calibration procedure every time. We would only use the probe tubes for one person, then throw them away. After the calibration, we hang the system devices from your ears and place the probe tubes in your ear canals. We are trying to get them within 5mm of your eardrum.

To do so, we would typically check the positioning visually; however, in many modern systems, they will auto check the positioning, so we don't have to do it visually. Once that is done, we play different test signals through the speaker to assess what is happening.

We will do this with no hearing aids in, with the hearing aids in and turned off and finally with the hearing aids in and turned on. The results are shown on our computer in a simple to read visual manner.

We can see clearly where the amplification is missing the targets if that is the case. Sometimes, the amplification might not be enough, sometimes and in individual ears, we may see that there may be too much amplification at one or more points.

You know what, sometimes it is bang on target. More often than not, in the last few years, it is more or less bang on target. Here's the thing though, we don't and can't know that for sure. So the fact that many modern hearing aids perform in the ear as they should. Is not an excuse not to undertake the test.

Again, anyone who says it is is speaking utter rubbish. I have heard many reasons for not performing probe tube measurements on hearing aid users. They are generally all utter and contemptuous rubbish. Dr Cliff Olson AuD (a rising star in US

Audiology and a strong consumer education advocate) has a couple of great videos on the subject on Youtube.

In one of those videos, he identifies and refutes each excuse. You can take a look at those excuses and his answers by searching Youtube for "DR Cliff Olson AuD: 5 WORST Excuses to NOT use Real Ear measurement". The key is that excuses, no matter what they are, are bullshit.

When Should it be Done?

The answer to that is when you are to full prescriptive level, that could be at the first fitting, or it may be later, let me explain. If you are new to hearing aids, most professionals will not fit you to your prescription level at the beginning.

You simply wouldn't be able for it. You would find it uncomfortable and loud. To manage that, we fit you to a reduced level and over a varying (varying because it depends on the Patient) amount of time we would move you to the prescriptive level.

It is then that Real Ear Measurement should happen because it is then that we have reached the best possible amplification for your hearing loss. Therefore, that is the time to test the outputs in the ear. If you are an existing user of hearing aids buying a new set of hearing aids, well then we might fit you to prescription immediately. If so, well then the process should be done at the fitting.

Over the years, and as your hearing aids get older, we should perform the measurement again. Doing so allows us to ensure that your hearing aids continue to hit the targets you need.

The Best Possible Outcome

If I am committed to delivering the very best possible outcomes for my customers, I need to undertake some sort of probe tube measurement, be it REMs or Live Speech Mapping. It is only then that I can be confident that I am delivering what you need for the best possible outcome. In some cases, even after doing it, there can still be problems.

Hearing and hearing ability is unique. Sometimes people with treatable hearing losses have problems understanding speech in noise no matter what we do with their hearing aids. The problem is a function of an underlying problem in the hearing area of the brain, and no matter how well we fit the hearing aids, they may struggle to help.

Here's the thing though, we, and by that I mean the professional and you the user, will never know that is the case unless we have clear and irrefutable evidence that the hearing aid is performing at it's best. Undeniable proof that it is doing what it should in your ear canal. The only way to gain that conclusive evidence is through probe tube measurements.

I echo Cliff Olson when he says "I find it sad that some hearing care providers feel the need to fabricate excuses as to why they don't feel the need to perform Real Ear Measurement." We have known for years that all the studies support it as a best practice.

Best Practice guidelines indicate that probe tube measurements are the Gold standard for hearing aid verification and validation.

Find A Provider Who Does

It is my best advice to you, knowing what I know, after studying the studies available, and indeed through my own experience fitting hearing aids, that you need probe tube measurements as part of your hearing aid journey. It is my best advice to you to find a hearing care provider who does offer them when you are purchasing hearing aids. Ask any provider you deal with, do they provide probe tube measurements, if they say no, tell them you will go somewhere else.

The Follow-up Visit

Your first follow up visit is an important time for you and us. We want to know how you have been doing and how the hearing devices worked for you. We will ask you about your listening experiences with the devices and how you have been wearing them. Be prepared to give us an update on how you have got on in all the different listening situations you have experienced.

The questions we ask will cover how you did in noise, your perception of loudness, clarity, any discomfort, etc. Tell us everything; we want to know, we want to understand how you got on. It is worthwhile for you to keep a notebook or diary during the early period so that you can keep track of how you are getting on. A journal can be invaluable for us because you write down the information as it happens.

Fine Tuning

It is not unusual for fine-tuning of your hearing aids to be needed, sound is a very personal sense. To one person rock is sweet music indeed, but to another, it is a racket. In the same manner, what is right for one person with hearing loss may often be wrong for others. During this time, you will also become accustomed to the hearing aids; this takes some time. Again, the time it takes differs from one to the other.

It may also take some time for you to get the best out of your hearing devices. While we restore normal levels of hearing, the processing centres of the brain take some time to adjust. It takes time for your brain to sort out this new sound information. This period is called the rehabilitation period; while initial improvements happen quickly, full rehabilitation can take up to a year.

Reinforcement of Information

At this visit, we will also take the opportunity to reinforce all of the information we have already given you. We will again discuss the hearing aids and their functions and talk about your clean and care routine.

Ask Your Questions

You will probably have many questions of your own at this stage, make sure you ask them. We have given you a large amount of information during your earlier visits. If any of it is still unclear to you, ask us to go over it again. Since your fitting, you may have new questions. We try our best to cover all of the information you need to know and to make sure you understand.

However, even we forget things from time to time, so ask any questions and that you think you need an answered. If you need it written down, ask us to do that as well.

Aftercare from here can vary, but once I get you to where I want you, I would see you on a regular scheduled six-monthly basis. Those appointments would vary from thirty-minute meetings to full-on hour sessions where I would re-test your hearing.

Telecare

We have discussed Telecare or remote care within our profession for a long time. It offers the opportunity to reach remote Patients, offering them the care they need without travelling long distances to be present.

The broader medical and healthcare profession is exploring telecare across the world in areas with dispersed populations, and access to hearing healthcare is spotty. However, hearing aid manufacturers have turned their attention to the concept to deliver better service to the people who wear their hearing aids.

Introduction of Telecare by Signia

The introduction of telecare by Signia was an exciting development. In essence, Signia introduced a system whereby your hearing professional could make limited fine-tuning changes to your hearing aids remotely through an iPhone app connected to your hearing aids. I liked the concept a lot, although many within the Profession were a little suspicious.

Expansion of Telecare by Resound

Resound went one step further with the launch of their 3D platform. They offered a complete remote fine-tuning capability to the Professional, again through an iPhone enabled app. I thought to myself; now you are talking.

Complete Real-Time Telecare

Signia, not to be outdone, expanded their telecare offering to offer full fine-tuning ability. They also incorporated the ability to make voice calls to the Professional within their telecare app. But they didn't stop there.

Face to Face Remote Meetings

They also incorporated video calling to the system, which means that Patients can have a remote, face to face meeting with their professionals for aftercare and fine-tuning.

Why Should You Care?

Telecare is evolving, and nearly every major hearing aid brand is either offering it right now or will offer it shortly. Again though, not every hearing aid user will be interested. But I believe that as hearing aid user demographics change, so will the uptake of telecare.

What it Will Do

Simply put telecare will make life easier for users and professionals alike. It will mean that a hearing aid user will not have to attend the office physically to have changes made. It will also mean that Professionals can vary the follow-up schedule. Perhaps including one or two remote sessions into the program.

Moving forward and as the technology changes and evolves, it could open up a different business model. I mean what if the hearing aid brands made remote fitting possible? That could mean that the online business model would be more effective. It could also mean a complete change to how we as Professionals work.

Complete Remote Care

For instance, how would you feel about a future where you bought hearing aids online and where fitted and cared for remotely by a call centre anywhere? I certainly don't think that would be palatable for everyone, but I can imagine some would be happy with that if the price were right.

With the advent of the COVID-19 pandemic, the debate around telecare has taken on new urgency. Most within the profession globally are now trying their best to get a handle on remote care. I think this area will just expand and become mainstream, even after we consign this vile little disease to memory.

Hearing Aid Pricing

In the first edition of this book, I stayed away from hearing aid pricing, mainly because it made no real sense to talk about it because it varied dramatically across the world. I still am not going to speak about individual prices here.

Because I simply don't know what they are. However, I am going to try and explain in detail how I reach my pricing and why it might differ dramatically across organisations. I am not justifying anything, mainly because I don't feel I need to, I am merely explaining.

On Hearing Aid Know we try and include price guides for the UK, Ireland and the US. They are aggregate price guides, just giving ballpark prices that we have been able to discover. If you are interested in one particular hearing aid and its price in your country, you could have a look at Know to see if we have listed it.

That is not a defence of hearing aid pricing. I know that pricing can be a touchy subject across the consumer world. It is an explanation of how I come to my pricing. You should use it as a gauge to allow you to understand if someone else price is providing value for money.

What Goes Into The Price?

We base the retail cost of a hearing aid on similar factors across every organisation. The elements are, cost of the device to the retailer, the cost of delivering the device to you plus profit. It is a relatively simple equation or matrix. If you were to judge the price of hearing aids at a retail level against the cost at the wholesale level, you would consider the difference extortionate.

However, it isn't a simple mark up, and you aren't just buying a product. You are purchasing a product and a level of service which includes multiple visits. That service is supplied by a professional who sets a price on his or her time and experience.

I am one of those professionals; I think my time, knowledge and knack for making hearing aids dance is worth money. I am also a special person who should be much loved, my Mammy has told me so, so it must be true.

Let's Break Down the Price

Cost of devices (varies by technology level obviously and by any agreed discount levels)

The hearing test itself which is at least one hour (in the UK and Ireland this is often free, but if you buy the hearing aids it is kind of bundled into the price)

The fitting of the hearing aids, an appointment which usually takes at least forty-five minutes if not more.

Initial follow up visits, I like to do at least two during the first month. If at the second follow up appointment, I am not happy with the progress; I will schedule at least one more for two weeks later.

Ongoing service calls, there is some debate about how often this should happen, many feel calling you back once a year is enough, I generally like to see my customers every six months. Some people would call that overkill, but I want to do it.

For some Patients, a six-month visit is imperative; for others, twelve-monthly visits would probably be excellent. The issue for me is that I don't know which is which until I have some experience with them.

Undertaking six-monthly appointments make me feel comfortable that I am heading off any problems before they happen. These ongoing callbacks will continue until the hearing aids die, which will be for at least eight to ten years probably.

Occasional drop-in visits, Geoff they stopped working, you forgot to change your wax guards, oh yes sorry about that, how are the kids? Happens all the time, sometimes it isn't just wax guards.

That is Not Justification

I am not trying to justify prices here; I am merely trying to explain what goes into my assessment of the price I charge. I will probably spend at least twenty hours with a customer during the lifetime of a hearing aid, and I think my time and expertise is worth money. It is as simple as that.

I also have business expenses to cover, light, heat, a receptionist, equipment costs rent and rates etc. These things all affect the price I set for hearing aids. Is my retail price the same as others? Maybe, maybe not, however, I feel that the price I charge is commensurate with the level of care, attention and experience I provide.

The key here is that I have carefully made you aware of what I provide for the price I will charge. So you are very clear about what you are getting for the price I charge. What you need to understand is that what I offer may not be replicated by another provider. **That is your job to both understand and assess**.

Will a corporate business or another independent dispenser supply you with the same level of care and attention? Will their Dispenser have the same professional experience and expertise? If the answer is yes, well then you are assessing like for like.

There has been much talk about the greed of professionals, in particular in the United States. I can't comment on it because again, I don't know what the prices are or what the price includes. I also don't know what a professional considers is an excellent hourly rate over there.

If you are in the United States and looking for hearing aids, I think you can probably make a better assessment of that. The key learning I want to pass to you here is to understand what the price you pay includes, because if you know that implicitly, you will be able to make an educated assessment of the benefit to cost ratio.

The last thing I will say is that just because it is cheaper, doesn't mean it is the same. Always understand the broader picture and be sure of precisely what you are getting for the price you are paying. Always, always, get it in writing.

Changing Prices Internationally

Hearing aid prices have been changing globally over the last few years. There is downward pressure on prices across the world that is mainly driven by low price sellers. In essence, many of these are internet-based sellers that have no staff. What they do is generate leads that they pass onto private practices.

This practice forces the professional to either sell the devices that you are interested in at a price dictated or to switch-sell you to something else. Many national businesses have also reduced their pricing based on the model that they are delivering. For instance, some in the UK and Ireland probably have some of the lowest pricing available.

That realise that pricing through their business model, which in essence is a conveyor belt. Get them in, get them fitted, and see them when you can. I don't agree with that business model, but hey, it works for them, and there are plenty of people who buy from them.

Do those people buy from them a second time? Of that, I am not sure, but I regularly have their customers come to me for help. I generally tell them to go back and demand help, which is what they paid for.

Experienced users of hearing aids tend not to base their buying decisions on price, although of course, price is a factor. Experienced users are focused on service and care, while new users with little experience focus solely on price. This fact and the pricing of others has led to reducing hearing aid prices overall.

A good thing and a bad thing

For the consumer, this has to be seen as a good thing, right? Well yes and maybe no, but let me explain. There was room to reduce prices; however, I think that providers also need to be careful. If we reduce our rates so much that it makes no financial sense. The consumer is the one that will suffer. I said it earlier, just because it walks like a duck, quacks like a duck, doesn't mean it is the same duck!

It is a simple equation if my price does not cover service, I either don't give it, or I go out of business. It is as simple as that. I think the death of Independent hearing healthcare providers would be a terrible thing for the consumer generally. Independents do tend to act as checks and balances on the system.

So, how can I address the downward pressure on prices but also make sure that the prices I charge make financial sense for my business and the consumers I serve? Because as a business person, it is up to me to meet consumer demands.

Unbundled pricing

For many years there has been some debate within the profession about unbundling the pricing. By that, I mean setting out the price of the hearing aid and the price portion of the service and care. While some, particularly in the states, have gone down that route it is by no means widespread. I think it is an excellent idea because it implicitly informs a consumer what they are buying.

It could also open up the pricing arrangements; for instance, say you didn't think that you would need any more than one check-up a year because you are a confident, experienced user. I think I should be willing to deduct the costs of the extra check-up and set a price with you for any incidental appointments that arose.

There are some problems with using a system like this in the UK and Ireland because of the V.A.T. (Value Added Tax, like a sales tax) implications. It would mean hearing health providers who went down that route would have to begin to charge V.A.T. for the services they implicitly provide. It is something that we would have to consider.

For me, I think that is a winner for both of us, you get a deduction, and I am still covered for my time. I don't know how others in the industry feel about that, and I am not sure what you think about that, but I think it is something worth exploring. That is my opinion folks, for what it is worth, I don't know how others within the business feel.

Hearing Aid Manufacturers

There are many different hearing aid brands across the world, in particular in the US. There is also a host of new players becoming involved globally. However, the hearing aid space is dominated by the big six. They are the most prominent players in manufacturing globally and have the most significant market shares. Or at least it was.

The big six was made up of Widex, Starkey, Sivantos/Signia (formerly Siemens), GN Resound, Sonova (who own Phonak and Unitron, and finally William Demant (who own Oticon and Bernafon). However, Sivantos/Signia and Widex have merged to form WS Audiology. So we are left with the big five.

These manufacturers are the ones who dominate the global market, and they do so for a good reason. They offer some of the best hearing aids available today. Take it as read, if the hearing aids provided are not by the brands I have mentioned, they are also-rans or second brands.

In the next few pages, I would like to try and give you a high-level overview of who they are and what they offer. I will not cover them all though; I will explain a few. I will continue to separate Widex and Signia, because those brands will continue separately for many years to come.

Oticon

Danish Manufacturer, Talk About Brain Hearing

Oticon is a Danish hearing aid manufacturer; they are owned by one of the biggest corporations in hearing care called Demant. Oticon has been around for a very long time, and they are one of the biggest hearing aid brands globally.

In the past, their hearing aids have not been that great in fairness. However, a couple of years ago, they began to move ahead. Initially, they began to speak about Brain Hearing and how they designed their hearing aids to work with the brain. I could never really work out what that meant.

Anyway, shortly after, they introduced the Opn, that is when I got interested. The Opn is an astonishing hearing aid platform. Oticon launched a whole new way to handle directionality and therefore, process sound for the user.

I have used the Oticon Opn, and I have been very impressed, it is different from any other hearing aid that I have ever worn. The real difference is when you are in noisier situations, the difference between the Opn and other hearing aids is profound but subtle.

With standard hearings aids, the noise in a noisy situation is like a wall—a wall of sound with no nuance. You can hear the voices you need to, but the noise is in the background is like a wall. With the Opn, it is very different; there is a real nuance to the noise.

It seems that the user gets a more normalised sound picture. While this seems to be the case, it does not interfere with speech intelligibility. Generally, the conversation is effortless, and when people call you to get your attention, it seems easier to hear them.

Oticon says that this new strategy will deliver a more normalised sound picture to the brain and therefore tap into the brain's abilities to hear well in noise.

Oticon Hearing Aids

Oticon's latest hearing aid platform is the Opn S, but before I talk about it, I want to talk about some legacy stuff. It will become clear why, as we go.

In the past, Oticon used a somewhat confusing way to name their hearing aids, giving each level of technology a different name that covered a range of hearing aid types. For instance, the Ria, The Alta etc. They also offered six different levels of technology, two at each tech level. That meant the Ria and the Ria Pro were both entry-level hearing aids, but the Ria Pro was a bit more featured.

The introduction of the Opn range changed that though, they introduced the Opn in three levels of technology which use numbers to designate the level. The flagship device range was the Opn 1, the mid-level device range was the Opn 2, and the entry-level was the Opn 3.

While initially, the Opn was only available in behind the ear and receiver in canal devices. Oticon introduced Opn custom hearing aids in 2018. The custom hearing aids were Made For iPhone enabled, but only down to the In The Canal model, which is slightly larger than a CIC.

Oticon introduced the new Opn S in 2019, again, it was introduced in three levels of technology, the 1, 2 and 3 and only with the behind the ear and receiver in canal models. For the first time, they have also introduced a lithium-ion powered rechargeable receiver in canal device.

Is the Opn S worth buying? The Opn S is an upgrade of the original Opn. Yes, it is a little better than the Opn, but the real difference is probably the lithium-ion rechargeable option. In general and by now, most professionals will not be offering the original Opn, but if you find one that is, and they have discounted them enough, I would consider them.

Technology levels are always something that confuses prospective buyers; in essence, each technology level offers the ability to hear clearly in different situations. The premium range offers the best support in every sound situation. The entry-level will provide much less support.

That isn't necessarily a bad thing; maybe you don't need the support! A good analogy is a Sat-Nav on a car; you can have a shiny new car with a pretty and sexy Sat-Nav. However, if you only go to the local shops, it is neither much use to you or worth your extra money.

Hearing aid technologies are similar in concept, if you aren't very active socially, why would you want to pay for a level of technology that offers you the best support for hearing in complex sound situations? It is a lovely thing to have, but if you do not need it, why bother or be worried about it?

I explain technology levels later in the book; however, I just think it is worthwhile commenting here in our first introduction to manufacturers.

The Platform

Oticon's latest platform is called the Opn S. The platform uses the Velox S chipset, which they say offers a new level of processing power providing faster automatics, new highly sensitive detectors, and increased memory.

They say the new chipset is powerful enough to analyse 56,000 additional times per second than the original Opn. That translates to increased performance across both updated and new features.

The OpenSound Navigator, which is responsible for that unique way of processing sound works better than before. The new OpenSound Booster function in the accompanying app offers even more help in everyday noisy situations to those who need it most when they need it.

The new OpenSound Optimizer prevents feedback (annoying whistling). It allows the aids to deliver the optimal gain, providing more open fittings with no feedback.

A personal note on the OpenSound Navigator

Oticon introduced this entirely new way to handle sound inputs that is altogether different from any microphone strategy that has gone before. Without boring you with technical details, this feature allows you better access to sound from all around you while ensuring that you can still hear the conversation that you want to.

Both Steve and I have found this feature to be both very good, and dramatically different from anything we have tried before. Up until now, modern hearing aids have used a directionality method of attempting to pinpoint whom you want to listen to in a noisy place.

You could have your hearing aids set to focus straight in front of you, or you could widen that focus a bit to encompass more sounds, but it was really about narrowing the areas down you wanted to hear from and blocking out noise from elsewhere.

When using this strategy, the perception of the user was that they had a wall of noise behind them. They could hear the conversation they wanted to, but everything else was just that wall of sound. As I said, the new strategy gives a much more nuanced and normal sound picture.

For instance, when I wore them in a noisy situation, I could hear people having conversations behind or to the rear side. I didn't know what they were saying, and I didn't need to, but I knew it was conversations.

Opn S Hearing Aid Prices

We would expect the Oticon Opn S range to be sold at prices from £1200.00 to £2200.00 in the UK depending on the Practice and location. We would expect the range to be sold at prices from €1400.00 to €3000.00 in Ireland. We would expect the range to be sold at prices from $1500.00 to $3200.00 in the USA.

Opn S Hearing Aids

The Opn S is Made For iPhone enabled, and while the range is currently limited. I think Oticon will introduce custom Opn S hearing aids in late in 2020. We don't have any details on that, but if you occasionally take a look at the Hearing Aid Know website, we will announce the introduction and explore the features when it happens.

Opn S miniRITE

The Opn S miniRITE hearing aid model is a very discrete wireless slimline 'Mini-Receiver-In-Ear (miniRITE)' hearing aid using a 312 battery. Powerful fully featured and offering fantastic discretion.

Opn S miniRITE-R

The Opn S miniRITE-R is a wireless slimline Rechargeable 'Mini-Receiver-In-Ear (miniRITE)' hearing aid using a new lithium-ion rechargeable battery which offers 16 hours of use with five hours of streaming. The battery pack is easily replaceable in the clinic. The device also has a telecoil.

Opn S miniRITE-T

The sleek and discreet wireless MiniRITE-T features a telecoil and double pushbutton for easy volume and program control. It is powered by a 312 battery

Opn S BTE13 PP

The powerful and compact BTE13 PP fits hearing losses up to 105 dB SPL to benefit people with severe-to-profound hearing loss. The plus power solution features a telecoil, a tactile double pushbutton for easy volume and program control and a two-colour LED indicator to monitor hearing aid status for both users and caregivers.

Widex

Widex is a Danish Brand who has been around since the fifties. They were founded by two men who had left William Demant (Makers of Oticon and others), and they first manufactured out of a garage. Since that beginning, Widex has become famous for technical excellence and fantastic sound quality.

Widex has always followed its own agenda since its inception, they firmly base their devices in audiological research, and because of it, the strategies they use tend to be unique. For instance, they believe that the very soft sounds of speech are essential for understanding. So they amplify them to fit within your residual hearing.

That presents technical problems, and Widex was one of the only manufacturers to do it up to recently. That is just one example of what they have done differently. Widex were the first hearing aid brand to introduce active machine learning to their hearing aids with the introduction of the Evoke in 2018.

Widex Hearing Aids

Widex release their hearing aids on a platform which has four levels of technology and a family of hearing aid models at each level. It appears that this is the way they will continue to launch hearing aids in the future, so it is worth me explaining.

The premium level of technology in all of the new Widex devices has been the 440. The technology levels drop via the 330, 220 and finally the 110. Features differentiate the technology levels, the one with the latest and best Widex features is always the 440.

The Platform

Widex changed the way they designated their hearing aids with the launch of the Clear platform in 2009. Since then, they have named their hearing aid platforms using one name such as Clear, Dream, Unique, the Evoke and most lately The Moment. Within the platform is a full range of Widex hearing aid types at four levels of technology.

The Evoke is the last range of hearing aids from Widex. In 2020 they introduced the Moment platform. I spoke to some people earlier this year at Widex, sober, conservative people. Scientific people, not people prone to exaggeration or flights of fancy. While they did not tell me much, because they can't, they were using words like groundbreaking and paradigm shift.

While I would typically take such things with a pinch of salt, in this case, the people who are saying them made me think there was probably something in it. Now that they have introduced the Moment platform, I would have to say they were correct.

I will cover both the Evoke platform and the Moment platform here and probably for the rest of the year. It makes sense considering what is going on in the world, and the Evoke platform is still a fantastic set of hearing aids.

Widex Moment

They have introduced the Moment, and even with all of the madness, should be shipping in April. It will be available in the usual four levels of technology from the 440 down to the 110.

There are a few new things with the Moment range to discuss including the change in hearing aid type offerings and the lithium-ion based rechargeable hearing aids. The biggest thing is the massive change in the signal delay that is at the core of the signal processing strategy in the Moment

Every hearing aid suffers a delay in signal processing; in essence, it takes time to process sound and present it at the eardrum. While sound that enters the ear canal in a normal way doesn't, leading to an out of sync signal. If the signal delay is 11 milliseconds or over, it produces an intolerable echo. Under 11 milliseconds, the echo is still there but is tolerable, and eventually, the brain will blend it out.

That signal delay ensures that hearing aids sound like hearing aids. The brain perceives the delay, and the sound is abnormal. Over time, the brain normalises it to a large extent, but it is never what you would call natural.

No Delay

The Moment is the first hearing aid that offers no delay in signal processing. Something quite astonishing, to be honest. That is a game-changer, and without doubt, it is a paradigm shift in hearing aid sound.

The Moment offers zero delays, which means natural delivery of processed sound at the eardrum, which should translate to very natural sound experience. Widex say that the Moment is the most natural-sounding hearing aid ever produced, and technically it should be.

They have also introduced a new way to assess leakage of sound from the ear canal. This new strategy should offer an even more accurate understanding of what is happening in your ear canal with the aid inserted. The new system is called TruAccoustics, and it will ensure that the hearing aids are offering sound at an optimum manner in the ear. The feedback from early testers is outstanding.

The Headlines

The headlines of the launch include:

1. New platform offers three RICs and three ITEs at present
2. ZeroDelay sound processing, a real breakthrough
3. TruAccoustics, providing an even better fit
4. Lithium-ion powered rechargeable hearing aid
5. New updated Bluetooth radio which offers iPhone connection and Android connection in the future

I think the Widex Moment will go down as a device that changed hearing aids, just like the Widex Clear did in 2009 and the Widex Senso back when dinosaurs roamed the earth.

Widex Moment Hearing Aid Prices

We would expect the Moment hearing aid range to be sold at prices from £1000.00 to £2200.00 depending on the technology level in the UK also dependent on the Practice and location. We would expect the range to be sold at prices from €1100.00 to €3000.00 in Ireland. We would expect the range to be sold at prices from $1400.00 to $3200.00 in the USA.

Widex Moment Hearing Aids

The Moment platform will come in six hearing aid types across the usual four levels of technology from Widex, the premium

440, upper mid 330, lower mid 220 and the entry-level 110. Initially, there will be no Behind The Ear hearing aids available. However, that will change later this year.

As I said, six hearing aid models, three Receiver In Canal hearing aid models and three In The Ear hearing aid models. The Receiver In Canal models are the RIC-10, which is the updated replacement for the Passion. The RIC 312D which replaces both the Fusion and the Fusion 2 and the new mRIC-R D which is a lithium-ion powered Mini Receiver In Canal hearing aid.

The RIC-10 (runs on a size 10 battery) is a very discreet device and the Passion it is based on was amazingly popular. The device is tiny, so it doesn't have a telecoil onboard, nor is it Bluetooth enabled. Although, they are wireless and can access loop systems and streaming audio from other sources via a Dex.

The RIC-312D (runs on a size 312 battery) is the same size and shape as the Fusion and Fusion 2 which it replaces. It is a hugely versatile RIC that will cover hearing losses down to severe to profound. It has a telecoil onboard and the new upgraded Bluetooth radio that is Made For iPhone compatible and ready for Made For Android.

The new mRIC R D is a very discreet lithium-ion powered rechargeable RIC. It is a very versatile RIC which will cover hearing losses down to severe to profound. It offers a telecoil and the new Bluetooth radio which provides a direct connection to iPhones and other Apple products and is ready for Made For Android. Widex say that it is the smallest rechargeable RIC available on the market. The device looks about the same length of the RIC 10 but broader at the bottom.

The device offers twenty hours of use with one charge and sixteen hours of use with streaming. I like the rechargeable devices, but I think I will reserve judgement on the charger. I can't say for sure, but it looks more like a desk type charger like the system Oticon uses rather than a multi-functional on the go charger like the one ReSound uses for the Quattro.

That is a pity, to be honest with you, apart from Signia with the charger for the Styletto Connect; no one else is innovating on the charger unit for their rechargeable devices.

The three In The Ear hearing aids are the IM, the XP and the CIC. None of them has a telecoil, although they can access loop systems via a Dex. None of them is Bluetooth enabled although they are wireless and can connect to the Widex Dex accessories for streaming audio.

The IM is powered by a 312 battery and has a programme button as an option. It will cover moderate to severe hearing losses. A 312 battery powers the XP, it will not offer a programme button option, and again it will cover moderate to severe hearing losses. The CIC is powered by a size 10 battery, and it will not offer a programme button and again will cover pretty much the same hearing losses.

The absence of a programme button means that you will not be able to access any extra programmes unless you have a Remote Dex or use the Tonelink app on your smartphone.

Widex Evoke

The Evoke platform or E-Platform was the first-ever range of hearing aids with machine learning capabilities. Although, the machine learning feature is only available on The Evoke Fusion 2, which is the direct connection or Made For iPhone hearing aid.

In essence, it is one of the latest Bluetooth enabled hearing aids just like the Widex Beyond before it. Widex said that the Evoke began the era of intelligent hearing, where the quality of your listening experience will evolve in real-time and real life.

With machine learning enabled, the Evoke range will continue to learn from you (and millions of others) as you use them so that you will hear sound perfectly.

Widex new SoundSense Technology means that every time you use EVOKE hearing aids, they evolve in their function. That's why they call them the world's first smart hearing aid. Because when you (and others around the globe) personalise your listening experience, EVOKE learns from different situations and your inputs.

Widex then uses anonymous data from your changes to create a better listening experience for everyone. That means that the hearing aids you buy will be better tomorrow than they were today. Widex has already used the system to push out an update in functionality to Evoke hearing aids. How long they will continue to do so is anyone's guess though.

Widex Evoke Hearing Aid Prices

We would expect the Evoke hearing aid range to be sold at prices from £1000.00 to £2200.00 depending on the technology level in the UK also dependent on the Practice and location. We would expect the range to be sold at prices from €1100.00 to €3000.00 in Ireland. We would expect the range to be sold at prices from $1400.00 to $3200.00 in the USA.

Widex Evoke Hearing Aids

Widex has a full line of hearing aids in every family, so that means within the Evoke platform, they offer Behind The Ear devices (BTE), Receiver in canal Devices (RIC) and custom In The Ear devices (ITE). Those devices would include:

CIC-M: This is the smallest of the range of custom ITE hearing aids; it is a non-wireless micro completely in canal device using a size 10 battery.

CIC: This is a slightly larger custom ITE device; it is a wireless completely-in-canal device using again a size 10 battery

Custom: This is a newly introduced wireless hearing aid model, it is in between the CIC and the XP but it offers a lot more versatility. For the first time in a long time, these devices will offer physical controls which mean you can have a volume control or a programme button on them. Unfortunately, the device will not have a telecoil. They are run on a 312 battery which means longer battery life.

XP: The XP is for all intent and purposes a half shell type custom ITE device. It is a wireless in-the-ear device with a telecoil using a Size 312 battery

PASSION: The Passion has for many years been the smallest RIC hearing aid available, but it has lost that honour to the new Unitron Now. It is a wireless mini receiver-in-canal device which uses a Size 10 battery. The size does limit the device though; it has no telecoil or programme button.

FUSION: The Fusion is a larger wireless receiver-in-canal device; it comes with a push-button and telecoil and runs on a size 312 battery.

FUSION 2: The Fusion 2 is very like the Fusion, it is a larger wireless receiver-in-canal device; it comes with a push button and telecoil and runs on a size 312 battery. The difference is that the Fusion 2 is a Made For iPhone hearing aid.

The Fusion 2 can also be fitted with a rechargeable system. Widex is the last hearing aid brand to use the Z Power silver-zinc rechargeable system. Just lately, they have announced an upgraded version of it. Stay away from it, it is more trouble than it is worth.

FASHION: The Fashion was introduced a couple of years ago as a replacement for the original 9 and 19 configurations, it is wireless slimline power BTE which can be used with a thin tube or a standard tube and mould. It has a volume control and telecoil and is powered by a size 312battery.

Fashion Power: Pretty much exactly the same as the Fashion but designed to deliver for profound hearing losses.

FASHION Mini: The Fashion Mini was introduced in 2016 as a replacement for the original M configuration; it is wireless slimline mini BTE which can be used with a thin tube or a standard tube and mould. It is an exceptionally discreet BTE and is powered by a size 312battery. It offers the discretion of a RIC with the reliability of a BTE, an excellent combination.

Each of these hearing aid types would be available in the four levels of technology available from Widex within the Evoke platform. For instance, there is a Widex Evoke CIC-M 440, 330, 220 and 110 available.

Phonak

Phonak is a Swiss manufacturer of hearing aids who are owned by Sonova. They are one of the biggest hearing aid manufacturers in the world. They have been manufacturing hearing aids for over half a century and provide their devices in over 100 countries around the world. While they were once known for hearing aids for children, they have become known for leading hearing aid technology that is suitable for all.

Phonak is rated as one of the best hearing aid manufacturers around today, and they consistently work to improve their technology. Any experience I have had with Phonak hearing aids has been a good one and customers are always impressed with the benefit they provide.

Phonak Hearing Aids

Phonak do things a little differently than the other manufacturers when it comes to naming their hearing aids. They do introduce their hearing aids as easily identifiable platforms, and they do use numbers to signify technology level. However, they split their hearing aid types with different names.

For instance, a flagship or premium range hearing aid from Phonak will use the number 90 while a basic level hearing aid will have the number 30 in the name. The four levels of technology are the 90, the 70, the 50 and finally the 30. Their BTEs are called Bolero, their ITEs are called Virto, and their RIC / RITEs are called Audeo. They also offer super power hearing aids named Naida.

The Platform

There are currently still two Phonak hearing aid platforms available. The Belong platform is Phonak's last full range hearing aid platform. While the new Marvel platform was only available in the Audeo range (RICs/RITEs) and Bolero range (BTEs). They have now launched the Virto (In The Ear Models) and the Naida (Super Power models) Marvels.

I would imagine that it will mean that the Belong platform will fade away over 2020. The Marvel has caught the imagination of both the public and the professionals who dispense hearing aids equally. I have worn a set, and I have been extremely impressed with them.

Before I go further, I need to explain something. The chip that runs the Marvel, is, in essence, the same chip that runs the Belong. They have upgraded the software on the chip and added brand new Bluetooth connectivity.

The reason I bring this up is that they have introduced the Virto Marvel. Some of those devices do not have that Bluetooth connectivity. In essence, you will be buying a Belong, with some upgraded features. It is something you need to know and consider.

Made For Any Phone

While most of the hearing aid brands went for Made For iPhone hearing aids, Phonak decided that they would go a different way with their mobile phone connectivity. They chose one that would give them a direct connection to any mobile phone.

Phonak relied on the traditional Bluetooth protocol, which offered tremendous benefits.

It meant that any hearing aid they produced would be technically able to connect to any Bluetooth enabled device, not just phones. That strategy also presented real technical difficulties. The first Made For Any Phone hearing devices (The Audeo B-Direct) did not offer stereo audio streaming of phone calls or any other audio. It also ensured that Phonak's quite famous ear to ear features did not work.

A New System, No Limits

The new Marvel platform does not have any of those limitations. The Marvel allows users to experience stereo streaming audio from any Bluetooth enabled device, that includes most mobile phones available, computers, even some modern TVs.

Marvel users can have that audio streaming with the full benefits of Phonak's ear to ear features (Binaural Voice Streaming Technology BVST for short). That all means an excellent new hearing aid platform with no limitations.

Fully Featured Hearing Aids

As I said, these hearing aids aren't de-featured in any way. They include all of the latest Phonak features, including their much-celebrated ear to ear features. They also have a brand new sound management system, which they call Autosense 3.0.

It recognises and automatically adapts to precisely match more listening situations than ever before. Autosense 3.0 also classifies streamed signals and will adjust how it works to help you to hear the way you should.

Multi-functional and Feature Rich Hearing Aids

These hearing devices are hugely multi-functional and feature-rich. The Marvel contains probably every single one of the current headline features in the hearing aid world, and they have even thrown in some new ones, here's the quick list:

- Stereo Bluetooth streaming: Stereo streaming from any Bluetooth enabled device, that means iPhone, iPad, laptops, computers, Macs, Android phones, Windows phones, hell any Bluetooth-enabled phone.
- Real Hands-free calling in stereo: Like the Audeo B-direct, the Marvel offers true hands-free calling from Bluetooth-enabled phones and VOIP services like Skype, except, to both hearing aids.
- TV Streaming: Marvel can stream directly from Bluetooth-enabled TVs, and can also stream from the Phonak TV Connector accessory.
- Rechargeability: They say both Marvel rechargeables will deliver a full day of hearing aid use from a single charge.
- Remote adjustments: Marvel hearing aids can be adjusted remotely by your hearing expert.
- New App Eco-System: Brand new apps to make life easier and engage the consumer in the process.
- RogerDirect: This is fascinating; for the first time, users will be able to stream from Roger devices directly to their hearing aids (won't happen until late 2019).
- Full Phonak Feature Set: The Marvel will offer comprehensive and up to date inter-ear features.

Stereo Bluetooth streaming

Marvel will directly stream stereo audio from any device capable of streaming audio via Bluetooth. That includes almost any device you can think of. You can connect it directly to your Android phone; you can connect it directly to your Mac Book or Windows laptop.

You can even connect it directly to any Bluetooth enabled television although you shouldn't. It will eat your batteries. That is pretty amazing, that is a direct connection without any streamer. The quality of streaming audio is excellent; the sound is full and bright. Music is warm and full, and phone calls are clear.

True Hands-Free Calling

The Marvel delivers true hands-free calling in stereo. You will hear your phone calls in both ears, giving you a better chance to understand the caller. Hands-free means you don't need to touch your phone. Your phone can be up to thirty feet away. You simply hit the button on your hearing aid to answer the call.

I loved this feature; there is a real feeling of freedom delivered by just touching your hearing aid to answer a call and chat away. My experience with it was that I never had any difficulties understanding what the caller was saying; however, in some noisy situations, they seemed to have some trouble with what I was saying.

More Than Just Audio Connection

The Bluetooth connection is being used for more than just audio streaming, though. They will also use that same connection for data exchange between the mobile phone and the hearing aids. This ability offers much more benefits for consumers and professionals alike. The data exchange is the core of the new ability to remotely fine-tune the hearing aids in real-time and for the user to give real-time day to day feedback with the new Hearing Diary.

RogerDirect

This system is worth mentioning; I used two RogerDirect devices, the Roger Pen and the Roger Select. I have to say; I was utterly and thoroughly blown away by their function. They were both genuinely fantastic in noisy, complex situations.

I warn you, they are expensive pieces of kit, but if you score higher than 15 on your QuickSIN (Quick Speech In Noise, discussed earlier), you need to consider kit like this.

The Roger devices are assistive accessories designed to give you the optimal opportunity to hear well in noise. They work exceptionally well, and they could be the difference between you being able to engage or not.

Up to now, using a Roger system was unwieldy at best, it involved you either adding special receivers to the bottom of your hearing aids or using a special streamer.

The new RogerDirect system eliminates that need with Roger devices. They stream their audio directly to Marvel hearing aids with the connectivity function. No ungainly receivers or streamers.

The Roger Pen

The Roger Pen looks just like a pen; it is a multi-functional rechargeable device that comes with a dock. The dock recharges the device and acts as a physical connection to sound sources such as your TV or stereo.

The pen has multiple smart microphones and a system that understands the physical aspect of the device. By that I mean if it is hanging around someone's neck, the device knows that and focuses on the voice above it.

If you are holding it and pointing it at someone, it knows it and focuses where you are aiming it. If you lay it on a table, it knows it and focuses all around.

No matter the aspect, it is continuously working to give a clear speech signal and cut down on background noise. It is truly effective at it, as well. My experience was outstanding.

As I said, unfortunately, this is a pretty expensive bit of kit, and the system can cost up to two grand in your favourite currency. That is on top of the cost of the hearing aids.

The Roger Select

The Roger Select is a discus type remote microphone. Like the Roger Pen, it has smart microphones and a system that understands the aspect of the device. This isn't a point and hold device, though. It acts as a remote microphone that you can hang around your companion's neck or a table microphone.

When you lay it on a table, it will automatically try to find the dominant speaker and deliver a clean speech signal. However, you can easily over-ride that by clicking on the Select to focus it in any direction.

Again, a fantastic if an expensive piece of kit. I have included them because they are outstanding. They are excellent devices if you need them.

The Hearing Aids

Let's take a look at the hearing aid types that are now available in the Marvel range.

Audeo Marvel Hearing Aids

The Marvel Audeo family is made up of five hearing aids of which two are rechargeable. The smallest traditional Zinc Air battery size is the 312. Below you can see a quick explanation of the devices and their expected availability.

The devices will be available in four levels of hearing aid technology as you would expect from Phonak. For the first time, Phonak has made the rechargeable devices available at every level of technology.

The Models

Audeo Marvel R: The Audeo Marvel R is Phonak's latest rechargeable Made For Any Phone hearing aid, it is quite discreet and we can use several receiver variations meaning it can cover a lot of hearing losses.

The device will connect directly to any Bluetooth enabled Mobile phone and will stream phone calls and audio in stereo.

Audeo Marvel 312: The Audeo Marvel 312 is a small RIC device which uses a size 312 battery, it is quite discreet and can be used with several receiver variations meaning it can cover a lot of hearing losses.

It doesn't have a telecoil although as always it is a wireless device. The device will connect directly to any Bluetooth enabled Mobile phone and will stream phone calls and audio in stereo.

Audeo Marvel 312 T: The Audeo Marvel 312T is a small RIC device which uses a 312 battery, it is still very discreet and can be used with several receiver variations meaning it can cover a lot of hearing losses.

This device has a telecoil. The device will connect directly to any Bluetooth enabled Mobile phone and will stream phone calls and audio in stereo.

Audeo Marvel 13T: The Audeo Marvel 13T is a RIC device that uses a size 13 battery. It is slightly bigger than the 312, but still pretty discrete. It can be used with several receiver variations meaning it can cover a lot of hearing losses.

The device has a telecoil, and will connect directly to any Bluetooth enabled Mobile phone and will stream phone calls and audio in stereo.

Audeo Marvel RT: The Audeo Marvel RT is a rechargeable RIC hearing aid which will have a telecoil. It can be used with several receiver variations meaning it can cover a lot of hearing losses. The device will connect directly to any Bluetooth enabled Mobile phone and will stream phone calls and audio in stereo.

Virto Marvel Hearing Aids

Phonak have now delivered the full Virto Marvel hearing aid range, and it includes the new Virto Black model that has received enormous attention. Phonak say that the Virto M range will continue to use the biometric calibration system, which takes your ear anatomy and hearing needs into account.

It identifies over 1600 biometric data points in and on your ear, and they use the unique calibration settings for each Virto hearing aid. In this way, Virto M can more reliably sense where the sound is coming from, thereby giving you access to a better hearing performance.

Using The Outer Ear

Phonak are the first and only hearing aid manufacturer to carefully map the outer ear to take advantage of its natural abilities. The outer ear naturally heightens some sounds while also helping us to identify the location of sounds.

They say that the process delivers a 2dB signal to noise ratio improvement. That means it will make the signal (what you want to listen to) 2dB higher than the noise. 2dB doesn't sound like much but combined with all the other strategies that Phonak use it will be a marked improvement.

Fully Automatic

The Virto Marvel hearing aids are fully automatic and run on their latest AutoSense OS™. However, not all of the Virto Marvels will offer that outstanding connectivity. The Virto M is available in four models, of which only two offer connectivity.

Again, as I said earlier, this is the Belong chipset with a software upgrade and fantastic connectivity. If you take the connectivity away, is it worth considering an upgrade? I think that is something you need to decide and I can't honestly advise you.

Four Levels of Tech

The Virto Marvel will be available in the usual four levels of technology, the 90, 70, 50 and 30.

While they may expand the types, the currently available Virto Marvel hearing aids are:

Virto M Titanium: The Marvel titanium is a very discreet and robust device. The Titanium was the first hearing aid device to use medical-grade titanium to form the custom shell. While this alone is innovative, Phonak used the properties of the metal to ensure that they can offer discreet custom hearing aids to more people than ever. It is very discreet, may not be suitable for everyone and has no connectivity.

Vitro Black: This is the device that was raved about at CES (Consumer Electronics Show) 2020. It is an In The Canal/Half Shell (depends on the ear canal really) custom hearing aid powered by a 312 battery and it comes with dual microphones. It also offers the full benefits of that outstanding connectivity, including the RogerDirect system.

Virto M-10 NW O: This is the smallest of the devices. The 10 means it takes a size 10 battery, NW means no wireless, so you miss out on all of the features for which you need wireless connection. O stands for omnidirectional, which means that you don't get the benefits associated with dual microphones.

Virto M-312 NW O: This device is a slightly larger mini-canal device with a 312 battery, unfortunately, to get the discretion, you lose out on the wireless features, and you only get omnidirectional microphones.

Virto M-312: This device is a more substantial aid that takes a size 312 battery. This device is the same as the Virto Blck, except it comes in the more traditional colours.

It is an In The Canal/Half Shell (depends on the ear canal really) custom hearing aid powered by a 312 battery and it comes with dual microphones. It also offers the full benefits of that outstanding connectivity, including the RogerDirect system.

Bolero Marvel Hearing Aids

The Bolero Marvel range is the latest range of Behind The Ear hearing aids from Phonak. It consists of just two hearing aid models, The Bolero Marvel M and the Bolero Marvel PR, which is a little strange. Both devices only cover hearing losses up to moderate to severe. Phonak would usually introduce a larger range of Bolero devices including a device that would cover severe to profound hearing loss. This time, they haven't, I think that means that we will see the Naida Marvel range of hearing aids introduced soon.

Bolero Marvel M: The Bolero Marvel M is a pretty discrete mini BTE with a multi-functional button, not unlike the button used on the Audeo. The M can be fitted with a slim tube (which you can see above) or an ear hook for traditional tubing and ear mould. The M will cover hearing losses down to 75 dB in the low to 95 dB in the high frequencies. That, of course, depends on configuration, with the slim tube fitted, that reduces to 80 to 85 dB in the high frequencies. The M has all of the features of the Marvel platform with a direct connection to any Bluetooth mobile phones and Roger devices. However, the M does not have a telecoil onboard, so a link to a Loop System is out. The device will be available in the four levels of technology, the 90, the 70, the 50 and the 30

Bolero Marvel PR: The Bolero Marvel PR is slightly larger than the M, but it is still relatively discrete. It uses the same multi-functional button as the smaller M. The PR is a lithium-ion powered rechargeable hearing aid can be fitted with a slim tube (which you can see above) or an ear hook for traditional tubing and ear mould. The PR will cover hearing losses down to 80 dB in the low to 100 dB in the high frequencies. That, of course, depends on configuration, with the slim tube fitted, that reduces to 70 in the low and 90 dB in the high frequencies.

The PR has all of the features of the Marvel platform with a direct connection to any Bluetooth mobile phones and Roger devices. It also has a telecoil onboard so it can be used to connect to a Loop System. Phonak say that you will get a full day of use out of one charge and use time is similar to the Audeo. The device will be available in the four levels of technology, the 90, the 70, the 50 and the 30

Naida Marvel Hearing Aids

Phonak has just recently introduced the new Naida Marvel range. While the older Naida ranges offered plenty of choices, the latest Marvel range only comes in one model. A Super Power Behind The Ear hearing aid. That feels a little strange, to be honest with you.

I don't know if it is that Phonak have become victims of their success and they just can't manufacture more models at the minute. Or if Phonak has decided the future for Naida is one focuses product.

Even the fact that it is merely available in a Super Power type is a little fascinating. There is no Ultra Power and indeed no rumour about one to come. In fairness to Phonak, the Super Power is almost as powerful as there older Ultra Power was. However, it still seems odd.

Naida V SP: The new Naida V SP is quite a small superpower hearing aid. It runs on a size thirteen battery and can be fitted with a power slim tube and tip which offers real discretion. The device can also be fitted with a standard thick tube and mould configuration. The SP runs on a size thirteen battery which accounts for that smaller size.

Starkey

Starkey is an American hearing aid manufacturer who became famous for their custom hearing aids. They produced very discreet custom hearing aids at a time that others had problems doing it. They are exceptionally popular in the States, and there are more than a few providers in the UK that use them as a primary manufacturer.

I don't like them, their hearing aid technology has always seemed okay, but I had a lot of problems with reliability. So much so that I just stopped using them.

Starkey Hearing Aids

Starkey is similar to the other manufacturers when it comes to naming their hearing aids. They do introduce their hearing aids as easily identifiable platforms, and they do use numbers to signify technology level. However, they too divide different hearing aid types with different names.

For instance, a flagship or premium range hearing aid from Starkey will use the number i2400 while a basic aid will have the number i1600 in the name. Their full line hearing aid offering is called Muse IQ, their IIC hearing aids are called SoundLens Synergy IQ and their Made For iPhone hearing aids are called Halo IQ.

The Platform

Starkey has a few hearing aid platforms floating around right now; they have a new platform called Livio Edge and two slightly older ones called the Livio and the IQ platform. The Livio Edge and the Livio AI are of real interest to me. I think they represent the future of hearing aids. Starkey has used the tagline "Welcome to the revolution".

Believe it or not, I am inclined to agree with them; the Livio Edge and AI before it, represent a revolution in hearing aid functionality. Are they any use as hearing aids? Haven't a clue, I have yet to experience them. Let's discuss what they are doing.

Livio Edge

Starkey announced the introduction of a lithium-ion powered Bluetooth, In The Ear hearing aid, among other things at their big Expo 2020 event in Vegas. That is a very big deal, rechargeable and Bluetooth in a custom product, the very first of its kind.

They said the device would be available on their new Livio Edge platform. The platform offers rechargeable custom models, three Receiver In Canal models of which one is rechargeable and a Behind The Ear model available in one premium technology level.

In The Canal?

They introduced the Edge AI platform in late February. It is available in an ITC (In The Canal) and ITE (In The Ear) device among others. Both the ITC and the ITE will be rechargeable. Both look like dual-mic custom devices with a push button. The faceplate seems to be raised in the middle with what I would assume are charging contacts.

Made For iPhone, Made For Android

The devices are Bluetooth enabled and will offer a direct connection to both iPhones and some Android 10 phones. That means direct audio streaming and call audio from those phones without any intermediary streamers.

Lithium-ion Powered

Making a custom hearing aid rechargeable has been technically difficult, the main issue has really how are you going to charge it. Starkey has solved the problem and this will be the first-ever lithium-ion powered custom hearing aid. They say the lithium-ion cell will give you 23 hours of battery life between charges.

Edge Mode

They discussed a new AI (artificial intelligence) powered Edge Mode during the presentation. They say that you can use the Edge Mode when you are in very complex sound situations to give you crisp, clear hearing. They said that crisp sound is delivered with a short burst of power when you need it most. It makes me wonder a little about the strategy.

They have said it is AI-powered adaptive tuning for the situation; the mention of a short burst of power makes me wonder about power use. It is just nerdy interest, but I wonder do they commit a higher level of power output to control the feature. If they do, it will be interesting to see what it does to battery life.

A Health-Focused Concept

Since the introduction of the Livio AI, it has been evident that Starkey sees the future of hearing aids in the broader health-focused concept. For want of a better description, let's call it a healthable device. The announcements of new apps, including the Thrive Care App and the Balance Builder App, just confirms and widens this strategy.

They have designed the Thrive Care App to allow caregivers or loved ones to keep track of a loved one's physical activity and social engagement. It makes a tremendous amount of sense; it will allow older hearing aid users to continue to live an active independent life while providing peace of mind for care providers.

Starkey has focused on falls before, and their Livio AI device will send out fall alerts when the hearing aids detect the user has taken a fall. Hearing loss is firmly linked to the risk of more falls. They designed the new Balance Builder app to help improve balance, stability, strength and gait. It guides the user through balance exercises and workouts, based on head movements detected from sensors in the hearing aids.

Blurring The Lines

Starkey has been blurring the lines between Hearables and Hearing Aids for a while now. The introduction of the lithium-ion powered Bluetooth ITE (In The Ear) device certainly does that. I think it is the first device from the hearing aid industry that can be firmly called a Hearable.

Livio Edge AI Hearing Aids

The range is made up of two rechargeable In The Ear hearing aids. The ITC and the ITE. A larger Receiver In Canal hearing aid, that comes in both rechargeable version and a non-rechargeable version and a mini RIC. It also offers a Behind The Ear hearing aid model.

The ITC is the smaller of the custom hearing aids and depending on the ear canal, and ear size could be an ITC or a half shell hearing aid. The ITE is a full shell model.

The rechargeable RIC and larger RIC are certainly not colossal hearing aids; they are relatively discreet on the ear. The mini RIC is quite small on the ear, while the BTE is larger, it is still a relatively discreet device.

Livio AI Hearing Aids

For the first time we have a hearing aid with built-in sensors, health tracking, fall detection and it translates 27 languages in real time. That's pretty revolutionary.

A hearing aid with hearable functionality

Starkey had teased the launch of the Livio AI for the longest time. They were talking about them mid-2018, but time dragged on with no sign. Eventually, on the 20th of March 2019, they had the UK launch in London which I attended.

The device has been a long time coming, and the outline of the functionality has excited a lot of people, I included. I believe the device represents a huge move forward within hearing aids. While I have heard a few people say that the broader functionality is just ancillary, I don't agree. I think the features are core to the devices and the users that they are designed for.

They Say Sound is Core

I have heard it said several times that sound quality is the real core focus of hearing aids, and that, of course, is true. Up to recently, Starkey wasn't famous for sound quality, although that changed slightly with the launch of the Muse.

Starkey says that the Livio AI represents their very best sound quality yet and they have introduced some new sound processing features to drive that. Of course, they would say that, however, I listened to the devices at the launch briefly and they sounded pretty good.

Of course, that is as artificial as it gets and by no means can be seen as putting them through their paces.

Binaural Communication

I was amazed to find out that Starkey had not been using binaural compression before. I mean it was first introduced by Widex almost ten years ago, and everyone uses some form of it now.

Anyway, Starkey is finally using binaural compression. They leverage the communication between two Livio AI hearing aids to produce a more natural sound, preserve the natural sound cues and to drive a better experience in noisy situations. That communication also allows them to re-produce inter-aural level differences, which will enable you to localise sound better.

That in itself should help you to separate speech and noise a little better in noisy situations. As I said, I had a brief listen to them through headphones, the location was pretty loud, and they sounded pretty good. It wasn't an authentic experience by any means, but with the limited, slightly artificial setup, they seemed okay.

Spatial Speech Enhancement

Starkey says that their new speech enhancement system will deliver a 10% reduction in cognitive effort in noisy environments and a pretty astonishing 80% reduction of noise. An 80% reduction against what is pretty unclear though.

Transient Noise Reduction

They have introduced a new system to handle transient or impact noises. The system identifies and reduces those noises quickly, which means a slamming door or dropped cutlery on a tile floor will not be as irritating.

Bluetooth Hearing Aids

The Livio AI are Bluetooth hearing aids, and they now will provide audio streaming and streaming of phone calls to the iPhone and select Android devices.

The Features

The feature set of these hearing aids is what sets them apart as innovative devices, here is a rundown:

- Translation in 27 languages
- Amazon® Alexa connectivity
- Rechargeable option
- Fall Detection and Alerts
- Heart Rate Measurement
- Voice-to-text Transcription
- Natural user interface with tap control
- Self Check for hearing performance
- Thrive Virtual Assistant, built on Google Assistant

Translation in 27 languages seems perhaps a little strange, but when you consider that older adults are exceptionally likely to travel, it starts to make sense. Starkey says that one of the core beliefs they have is that they enable communication, with live translation of different languages, they are doing that.

Health Monitoring

The Livio AI offers relatively decent health monitoring opportunities, while it monitors activity and now heart rate, it also monitors socialisation and how much time is spent engaging with people. The Thrive App uses all of this to give its scores.

Thrive app and Livio AI hearing aids

They provide the health monitoring element of the Livio AI via the Thrive App. It offers two measurements that both deliver the possibility of a score of 100 points. It focuses on a Body score and a Brain score.

They calculate the body score through a combination of activity, steps and overall movement. This information is tracked daily and accessed easily in the Thrive app. As I said, a daily score of 100 points is possible.

Cognitive Health

Starkey says that because of the critical connection between cognitive health and hearing health, Livio AI measures the brain benefits of wearing hearing aids. The metrics used to measure the Brain score include hours of daily use, social engagement and the tracking of active listening. Again the daily score of 100 points is possible.

Does it give you a score based on cognitive health? No, it doesn't, however, it gives you a clear idea about some of the things that we know promote good cognitive health and I think that is a good thing.

Because there is an important link between hearing loss and a lot of other co-morbidities like heart disease or diabetes. Enabling health tracking in a hearing aid makes perfect sense, I mean you wear them all day, so they are the ideal device to monitor activity.

Fall Detection & Alerts

Starkey is leveraging the sensors in the Livio AI to detect falls, and they have set up a system in the Thrive App that allows an alert to go out to up to three different designated contacts. I honestly think that this is a stroke of genius, I have said for many years that hearing aids could be the ideal platform for the monitoring of activity and health of older people, ensuring that they can lead independent lives for longer.

This system represents a big part of that concept. When you hear the figures (from National Council On Aging) relating to falls for older people, it begins to put the benefit of this feature in perspective:

- Every 11 seconds an older adult is treated in an emergency room for a fall
- Every 19 minutes an older adult dies from a fall
- $67.7 Billion in projected costs from fall by 2020

Older people fall down with alarming regularity and injure themselves, some of them die. The horrible thing is that some who die may have lived if help was quick enough to get to them. That's a hard pill to swallow, and I would imagine it would lead to great torture for a family.

The fall detection and alert system mean that if a Livio AI user falls, their loved ones should know about it instantaneously. I think that represents huge peace of mind.

The Self Check

The self-check feature in the Thrive app which will run a subroutine to check your hearing aids. It's a handy tool that allows you to be sure if you need to see your professional or the receiver is just blocked with wax.

Thrive Personal Assistant

You activate the Thrive Personal Assistant with a tap on the hearing aids and then simply speak your query. At present, the Thrive Personal Assistant handles your questions in two ways.

The AI in the app decides if your question is hearing aid related or a broader general query. If it is hearing aid related such as how do I turn the volume up, the query is handled locally within the app. If it is a broader query, like why is the sky blue?, the app passes it on to Google to answer.

The Models

The Livio AI is available three models, a mini receiver in canal, a rechargeable receiver in canal and finally a behind the ear device. They are suitable for mild to severe to profound hearing losses.

One Price Level

The Livio AI is only available at the premium price level. There are lower level Livio ranges but they do not have all the AI features.

SoundLens Synergy IQ

The SoundLens was the first of the modern invisible hearing aids. While they are not suitable for everyone, they seem to be pretty solid devices. Anyone I have ever come across wearing them has been very impressed with them. The Starkey SoundLens Synergy IQ comes in two styles:

Starkey SoundLens Wireless: This is a wireless (invisible-in-canal) device; however, it is only available in the premium range i2400.

Starkey SoundLens Non-Wireless: This is a non-wireless (invisible-in-canal) hearing aid and it is available at all tech levels.

Muse IQ

The Muse IQ range comes in a variety of styles:

Starkey Muse Mini BTE: This is a wireless BTE device, powerful but discreet traditional type BTE hearing aid. With rocker switch and telecoil (size 312 battery).

Starkey Muse BTE 13: This is a wireless BTE device, powerful but discreet traditional type BTE hearing aid. With rocker switch and telecoil (size 13 battery).

Starkey Muse Micro RIC 312t: This is a wireless mini RIC (receiver-in-canal) device, small, ultra-discreet but powerful hearing solution. With push button and multiflex tinnitus therapy (size 312 battery).

Starkey Muse RIC 312t: This is a wireless RIC (receiver-in-canal) device, larger than the micro RIC but still a discreet but powerful hearing solution. With push button and multiflex tinnitus therapy (size 312 battery).

Starkey Muse CIC: This is a wireless CIC (completely-in-canal) device, small, ultra-discreet but powerful hearing solution with optional telecoil depending on the size of the canal (Size 10/312 battery).

Starkey Muse ITC: This is a wireless ITC (in-the-canal) device, small, ultra-discreet but powerful hearing solution, with a telecoil (Size 312 battery).

Starkey Muse ITE: This is a wireless ITE (in-the-ear) device, a powerful custom hearing solution with a telecoil (Size 13 battery).

The Halo IQ

Starkey was the second manufacturer to introduce Made For iPhone hearing aids, and this is their third update of them. I have personally worn the Halo 2 devices at the premium range, and I have to say they were pretty good devices. Nice crisp sound, good connection to the iPhone and great power delivered through the app. The Halo IQ range is a Made For iPhone technology which comes in four styles, all of which are receiver in canal devices:

Starkey Halo IQ RIC 312: This is a wireless RIC (receiver-in-canal) device, small, ultra-discreet, but powerful hearing solution. With push button and multiflex tinnitus therapy (size 13 battery).

Starkey Halo IQ RIC 13: This is a wireless RIC (receiver-in-canal) device, small, ultra-discreet, but powerful hearing solution. With push button and multiflex tinnitus therapy (size 13 battery).

Starkey Halo IQ RIC 312 AP: This is a wireless RIC (receiver-in-canal) device, small, ultra-discreet but powerful hearing solution.

With push button and multiflex tinnitus therapy (size 13 battery). This device will cover very severe hearing losses.

Starkey Halo IQ RIC 13 AP: This is a wireless RIC (receiver-in-canal) device, small, ultra-discreet but powerful hearing solution. With push button and multiflex tinnitus therapy (size 13 battery). This device will cover very severe hearing losses.

Starkey Technology Levels

Starkey keeps to three levels of technology in its latest platform, the Premium i2400, the Advanced i2000, the Standard i1600. All of the hearing aids we have discussed here are available in those three levels.

Signia /Sivantos /Siemens

Siemens is a well-known German company, and their hearing aid division was one of the largest manufacturers of hearing aids worldwide. They sold their hearing aid division to a private consortium named Sivantos a couple of years ago. Sivantos have now changed the hearing aid brand to Signia. As I said earlier, Sivantos has now merged with Widex to form WS Audiology. However, the Signia brand will remain a factor for many years to come.

Signia Hearing Aids

Up to now, Signia has been similar to Phonak when it comes to naming their hearing aids. They do introduce their hearing aids as easily identifiable platforms, and they do use numbers to signify technology level. However, they split their hearing aid types with different names.

For instance, a flagship or premium range hearing aid from Signia will use the number 7 while a basic hearing aid will have the number 3 in the name. Their BTEs are called Motion, their ITEs are called Insio, and their RIC / RITEs were called Ace, Pure, carat and Cellion.

With the introduction of the new Nx range, the RIC / RITE naming seems to have changed. They appear to be calling the RICs Pure. They have also introduced a brand new RIC style that they are calling the Styletto. They also offer super power hearing aids named Nitro.

Telecare 3.0

This is an exciting development; Signia has made the Telecare service a live service. They were initially the first to offer Telecare with a limited fine-tuning option although Resound quickly followed with the launch of the LiNX 3D and their Remote Assist which had more functionality. Signia though rapidly expanded that fine-tuning option and added video calling to the system. Now they have enabled full live remote tuning with video support, which is a pretty huge breakthrough.

The new service means that you can set-up a video call with your hearing professional and explain the issue you are having in the situation you have it in. While you are connected, your hearing professional can tweak your hearing aid's settings live, and you can quickly assess if they are better.

The Platform

Signia's latest platform is the X range which is made up of only two Receiver In Canal hearing aids available in three levels of technology. The Nx range is still available, and It has a full range of model types including RICs, BTEs and ITEs.

Signia Xperience

The Xperience platform has several new features which many are excited about already. These are the first hearing aids to use motion sensors to change how they present sound. Let's take a look at both the devices and the features on offer.

New Model Designs, New App

The Xperience platform offers the new Pure 312 X (with optional T-Coil) and rechargeable Pure Charge&Go X hearing aids in three levels of technology. It also brings brand-new, all-in-one smartphone app offering greater convenience for users.

Those Motion Sensors

They say that the new platform introduces the world's first combination of advanced acoustic sensors with a built-in motion sensor. The hearing aids use the sensors to provide a complete analysis of the wearer's dynamic soundscape.

They say that the new system will allow for automatic adjustments between sounds in front of and all around the wearer for a more personalized listening experience. In essence, they are saying that they use the motion sensors along with their new analysis system to give users more access to the sounds around them without compromising on clarity.

Signia has been down this route before, but the original system used the sensors on a connected smartphone to deliver more data points to the analysis and processing system. Many hearing aid wearers have an active lifestyle that involves walking, cycling and even running. But no hearing aids take the movement of the user into account when the management system decides how to help them hear better.

It means that most hearing aids don't necessarily adapt well as the wearer moves around, especially so in complex sound environments. Signia say that the Xperience platform, built upon YourSound technology, was developed to fill this crucial gap and respond to rapid changes in the wearer's environment and their movement.

The Benefits

With the new YourSound technology, Signia Xperience hearing aids have access to more variables. It is a simple equation, the more you know about the variables in a situation, the better you can plan to deal with them. The same can be said about hearing aids that provide the best sound possible. Signia say that the built-in motion sensor will allow them to take into consideration how the wearer's movement affects their hearing in each situation.

They have introduced new technology which means the hearing aids no longer have to decide between focusing on what is directly in front of the wearer or in the general surroundings. The new system offers the wearer a more natural experience. They can continue benefit from the proper amount of frontal focus, while still being able to hear relevant speech from other directions.

Signia say the three key features of YourSound technology are:

- Acoustic-motion sensors for a complete analysis of each wearer's dynamic soundscape
- Dynamic Soundscape Processing for natural sound and speech from any direction, in any situation – even when moving
- Own Voice Processing (OVP™) for a natural sounding own voice

New Chipset, Smaller & More Powerful

The new Signia Xperience chip includes 80% more transistors and seven times the memory of the previous Signia Nx chip, while also being 60% smaller. As a result, the first two hearing aids on the platform, the Pure® 312 X and the Pure® Charge&Go X, are smaller yet more powerful than their predecessors.

Signia Xperience Hearing Aids

Pure 312 X: The new Pure 312 X offers a brand new design with a rocker switch powered by a 312 battery and an optional T-Coil. The receiver-in-canal (RIC) hearing aid also has Bluetooth® connectivity for effortless streaming of phone calls, music, and TV audio. There is an optional telecoil, and it is an inspired design.

While Signia has a fascinating add on telecoil that lives in a battery door, they have now designed a hearing aid case that has the telecoil built into it. It will merely be a case of changing the case (see what I did there?). Anyway, I think it is inspired. **If you purchase a 312 X and then decide at a later stage that you would like to sample the delights of modern induction loops, you simply get a new case put on your existing hearing aid.**

Pure Charge&Go X: The Pure Charge&Go X is a lithium-ion powered rechargeable RIC with Bluetooth connectivity. Signia say that the devices have 20% more charging capacity and are 16% smaller than the previous Pure Charge&Go Nx.

It adds up to a svelte and discrete device that offers better battery life even with streaming. Signia have introduced a new inductive charger with a lid to protect the hearing aids as they charge, something that many people had complained about. The charger also works as a dehumidifier and is designed to fit custom ear molds.

The New App

The new Signia app combines three existing Signia apps into one unified easy to use app that should meet user's needs, including:

- Providing wearers with direct support from a hearing care professional
- Remote control so the wearer can personalize their hearing experience
- Easy management of streaming accessories to fully enjoy phone calls, music, and TV

The introduction of integrated motion sensors to hearing aids offers a considerable amount of new possibilities. Signia is the first to do it, and they will learn a lot from experience. While they are using the onboard motion sensors to make the experience better, the information that Signia will learn from the system has even more promise for future breakthroughs and possibilities.

The next thing is adding a gyroscope sensor so that we can understand head aspect, that would allow us to understand listening intent better. The more you know about the variables in a situation, the better you can plan to deal with them. Signia has taken a significant step forward to a complete understanding.

Signia Nx Hearing Aids

Signia introduced the Nx hearing aids late in 2017, it added some outstanding new features.

Made For iPhone Bluetooth Enabled

The entire Nx range is Made For iPhone enabled hearing aids that offer a direct connection to Apple devices for audio streaming.

OVP, Own Voice Processing

Signia made a big deal of the OVP or Own Voice Processing at the launch, and these devices are the first hearing aids to process the user's own voice differently from everything else. In fact, they have dedicated a completely separate processor on the platform to facilitate that. They said that the strategy would increase the acceptance of a user's own voice dramatically.

I Second That

I have to agree wholeheartedly with that sentiment; the OVP feature is fantastic. My experience with it has been pretty jaw-dropping. In the article **Signia Pure 312 7 Nx Hearing Aids, Here is What You Need to Know**, I talked in more depth about the own voice processing feature and why it might be of interest to you. The pertinent statement here though is:

When I was fitted with the Nx I was fitted with closed domes; I thought this isn't going to work as I heard my voice explode in my head. Then, we went through the own voice training protocol (count from twenty-one until it is happy it knows your voice). The feature was turned on, and no more occlusion, just like that. I was a bit speechless (that doesn't happen very often). By no more occlusion I mean no more auditory occlusion, I wasn't caused any difficulty by my own voice.

For new users of hearing aids the sound quality of their own voice can be off-putting, but it is usually something that they get used to. However, as Signia point out, used to, does not mean happy with. This system promises to deal with the issue, and it does it exceptionally well.

Pure 13 NX: This device is an updated version of their Pure 13 BT, it offers the new system which separately processes the wearer's own voice. It comes with superior connectivity with direct streaming and the myControl App, which deliver personal control over the devices. The hearing aid has a rocker switch which allows programme changes and volume changes. It is IP68 rated and can be fitted with the four levels of receiver power, making it suitable for most hearing losses. Signia say that users will enjoy the longest wearing time in its class while streaming. It also has access to the full live remote support via TeleCare 3.0.

Pure 312 Nx: This device is a very svelte Pure (RIC) device using a 312 battery, again it offers the new system which separately processes the wearer's own voice. The hearing aid has a rocker switch which allows programme changes and volume changes. It is IP68 rated. It can also be fitted with the four levels of receiver making it suitable for most hearing losses. It comes with superior connectivity with direct streaming and the myControl App. It also has access to the full live remote support via TeleCare 3.0.

Motion 13 Nx: This device is a BTE device using a 13 battery, again it offers the new system which separately processes the wearer's own voice. It also comes with superior connectivity with direct streaming and the myControl App. It has access to the full live remote support via TeleCare 3.0. The device also offers the rocker switch for programme and volume control changes. That is a pretty versatile device which provides a telecoil option with the simple switching of the battery door. The device is IP67 rated for dust and moisture.

Pure 10 Nx: This ultra-small device is a very svelte Pure (RIC) device using a 10 battery, again it offers the new system which separately processes the wearer's own voice. The hearing aid provides no controls; however, paired with a remote control, you will have access to programme changes and volume changes. It is

IP68 rated. It can also be fitted with the four levels of receiver making it suitable for most hearing losses. It comes with superior connectivity with direct streaming and the myControl App. It also has access to the full live remote support via TeleCare 3.0. The device is available in three levels of technology.

Pure Charge N Go Nx: This device is a very svelte Pure (RIC) device which is powered by a Lithium-Ion rechargeable battery pack, again it offers the new system which separately processes the wearer's own voice. The hearing aid has a rocker switch which allows programme changes and volume changes.

It is IP68 rated. It can also be fitted with the four levels of receiver making it suitable for most hearing losses. It comes with superior connectivity with direct streaming and the myControl App. It also has access to the full live remote support via TeleCare 3.0. The device is available in three levels of technology.

Styletto Connect: The Styletto Connect hearing aid is a discreet Made For iPhone rechargeable device that offers coverage for mild to moderate hearing losses. It is attractive if different design and reminds you of high-end electronics as opposed to traditional hearing aids. The charger case is outstanding, and it delivers four extra charges for the devices, which means you can go away for a long weekend and forget your plug.

Like the original, the receiver is fixed in the hearing aid and can not be replaced in the clinic, it will have to be a factory repair job. That means that you will need to take care of it to ensure it doesn't fail. Generally, people do not take care of their receivers, we see them failing all of the time through user negligence. They get full of wax and moisture and die. The Styletto Connect is available in three levels of technology

Signia In The Ear Hearing Aids

Signia offers four In The Ear hearing aids in the Insio range, the Insio IIC, the Insio CIC, the Insio ITC and the Insio ITE:

Insio NX IIC: The IIC is a non-wireless invisible-in-canal hearing aid that uses a size 10 battery. The device is not Bluetooth enabled.

Insio NX CIC: The Insio CIC is a wireless completely-in-canal device that uses a size 10 battery. This device is not Bluetooth enabled.

Insio Primax ITC: The Insio ITC is a wireless in-the-canal hearing aid with a telecoil, and it can be ordered with a size 10 or 312 battery. This device is a Bluetooth enabled hearing aid.

Insio Nx ITE: The Insio ITE is a wireless full shell in-the-ear hearing aid with a telecoil, and it can be ordered with a size 312 or 13 battery. This is a Bluetooth enabled hearing aid.

GN Resound

GN Resound is another Danish hearing aid manufacturer with a long history. They are one of the top 5 manufacturers in the world and are renowned for innovation and continuously advancing technology. Since they began in the 1940s, Resound has continued to grow, but it is in the last 20 years, their innovation has pushed them to new heights.

They have had a lot of firsts over the years; their latest first was Made For iPhone hearing aids. They are still the only manufacturer that offers a full range of Made For iPhone (MFI) hearing aids including BTEs, RICs and ITEs.

Resound Hearing Aids

Resound are similar to the other manufacturers when it comes to naming their hearing aids. They introduce their hearing aids as easily identifiable platforms, and they do use numbers to signify technology level. Each platform would have a full range of hearing aids available

For instance, a flagship or premium range hearing aid from Resound will use the number 9 while a basic aid will have the number 5 in the name. Their latest full range hearing aid offering is called the LiNX 3D, although they have a newer limited range called the LiNX Quattro.

The Platform

As I said, Resound has a few hearing aid platforms floating around right now, the very latest full range of hearing aids is called the Linx Qattro platform. They also have the Enzo Quattro range Which is suitable for people with severe to profound hearing loss. They are all Made For iPhone and Made For Android hearing aids.

Linx Quattro Hearing Aids

Resound released the Linx Quattro range late in 2018. The Quattro works on an entirely new chipset from Resound that delivers a massive improvement in processing power and speed. Resound has used that chipset to full effect by completely re-designing their signal processing and the hearing aid features. They have also increased the bandwidth of the devices and the input range, which should translate to a cleaner, more natural sound.

Resound have redesigned the wireless radio though and they say that it is more powerful than ever before. That should translate into stable connection to the iPhone and hopefully Android phones when Android releases the new version.

Full Range, Three levels of Technology

The Quattro is available in a full range of models including Receiver In Canal models, Behind The Ear models and a plethora of In The Ear Models, most of which are Bluetooth enabled across three levels of technology. The devices are suitable for hearing losses from mild to severe to profound.

Made For iPhone, Made For Android

The Quattro was the first-ever Made For Android hearing aid available. Resound, and Google worked together to deliver hearing aid support to Android in 2019. It means that Quattro hearing aids (or at least most of them) will be able to receive streamed audio from Android phones directly, without the aid of an intermediary streamer.

Of course, there are caveats. The system will only run on Android phones using Android 10 with the right Bluetooth hardware. At present, that means the Pixel 3 and 4 range and the Samsung Galaxy 9 and 10 range. I think that will increase over 2020, but you will need to look up phone compatibility on the Resound website.

Here is a quick rundown of the Quattro:

- The devices will be available in three new technology levels
- The devices are available in a full range of types
- The devices are Bluetooth hearing aids
- The devices use a brand new chip platform
- The chip has 100% faster processing than 3D
- The chip has 100% additional memory over the 3D
- Resound are using a new way of handling directionality inputs
- They have introduced a redesigned wireless radio with extra signal strength
- They have extended the bandwidth of the devices giving extra high-frequencies
- They have increased their dynamic input range, calling it industry-leading
- The devices are available with a Lithium-ion rechargeable battery pack and without

- The rechargeable hearing device will deliver 24 hours of use with 50% streaming on a three-hour charge
- The Lithium-ion devices will deliver 30 hours of use without streaming on a three-hour charge

The Models

LiNX Quattro RIE-61 Rechargeable: The LiNX Quattro RIE-61 Rechargeable is a rechargeable direct connection, Bluetooth enabled or Made For iPhone hearing aid just like all the LiNX devices before it. Making it a rechargeable device makes a lot of sense, although they have used the chip upgrades to improve power consumption, a rechargeable option allows you the comfort of never having to worry about hearing aid batteries.

The battery life is also fantastic, they say that you will get 24 hours of life even if you are streaming for 50% of the time, that's pretty amazing. The device has no telecoil onboard, but if you pair it to a multi-mic, you can use the telecoil in that to stream to your hearing aids.

LiNX Quattro RIE-62: The LiNX Quattro RIE-62 is a traditionally powered hearing device using a size thirteen battery. It is slightly larger than the RIE-61, but it comes with an onboard telecoil. The new power management system should mean that the size 13 battery lasts even longer

LiNX Quattro RIE61: The LiNX Quattro RIE-62 is a traditionally powered hearing device using a size 312 battery. It is quite a discreet device, but it doesn't offer a telecoil. The new power management system should mean that the size 312 battery lasts even longer

IIC Invisible in Canal: This is a non-wireless invisible-in-canal device. It uses a size 10 battery. So it isn't a Made For iPhone device.

CIC W Completely in Canal: This is the first-ever Bluetooth enabled CIC, although, in my experience, it has been more an ITC size. It will connect to both iPhones and enabled Android phones for streaming of audio and phone calls.

ITC DW In The Canal: This is a slightly larger wireless Made for iPhone in-the-canal hearing aid. It uses a size 312 battery and can come with an optional telecoil.

ITE DW In The Ear: This is a larger full shell wireless Made for iPhone in-the-ear hearing with an optional telecoil. It uses a size 312 or 13 battery.

MIH W Microphone in Helix: Resound is the only manufacturers who offer this style of hearing aid, it is a non-wireless small microphone-in-helix hearing device. The microphone is attached to a wire that you place in the helix of your ear. It uses a size 312 or 13 battery and offers an optional telecoil.

BTE 67: This is a wireless Made for iPhone BTE that can be used with a thin-tube or standard BTE tubing and mould. This device has a push-button, volume control and telecoil. It uses a size 13 battery.

BTE 77: This is a wireless Made for iPhone BTE that can be used with a thin-tube or standard BTE tubing and mould. This device has a push-button, volume control and telecoil. It also offers Direct Audio Input, which means it will accept an audio boot. It uses a size 13 battery.

BTE 88: This is a wireless high-power Made for iPhone BTE. The device is fitted with a push-button, volume control and telecoil. It also offers Direct Audio Input, which means it will accept an audio boot. It uses a size 13 battery.

Enzo Quattro Hearing Aids

The Enzo Quattro superpower range has all of the features of the Quattro platform, including direct connection to both Apple and Android products. The range comes in two styles.:

Enzo Quattro 88 BTE: This is a wireless high-power Made for iPhone BTE. The device is fitted with a push-button, volume control and telecoil. It uses a size 13 battery.

Enzo Quattro 98 BTE: This is a wireless high-power Made for iPhone BTE. The device is fitted with a push-button, volume control and telecoil. It uses a size 675 battery.

Resound Technology Levels

As I said, there are three levels of technology in every Resound platform, in the premium ranges, the levels are the Premium 9, the Advanced 7, and the Standard 5.

Costco Hearing Aids

This is the first time I have included the Costco Kirkland range in the book. Considering many of my readers are from the US, it makes sense to do so. Costco is the most significant private provider of hearing aids in the USA. Costco introduced hearing aids a part of its offerings way back in 1989, and they have successfully built up their hearing centre network since then.

In general, the feedback on Costco provided hearing aids is generally good to mixed, just as it is from any other provider. Many Costco hearing professionals offer best-practice hearing care, including Real Ear Measurements. However, that doesn't seem to be consistent across all Costco hearing centres. The one thing that everyone agrees on is that the price of hearing aids at Costco is outstanding.

The Kirkland Signature 9.0 hearing aid range is made up of one Bluetooth enabled Receiver In Canal hearing aid at one premium level of technology. The hearing aid will fit most hearing losses because of the interchangeable receivers (speakers). The Kirkland Signature 9.0 can use four different receivers, which allows the hearing aid to cover hearing losses from mild to severe to profound hearing losses.

Kirkland 9.0 Hearing Aid

The device is an IP68 rated hearing aid with a multi-functional control button that is powered by a 312 zinc-air battery. It doesn't have a telecoil onboard. It is a Bluetooth hearing aid, and unlike other Bluetooth hearing aids, it offers a direct connection to any Bluetooth enabled cell phone.

Sonova manufactures the new Kirkland Signature 9.0, and they have built it upon the same hardware as the Phonak Marvel and Unitron Discover. You must understand that the Kirkland 9.0 is similar to these hearing aids but is not precisely the same.

Made For Any Phone

The Kirkland 9.0 uses the Sword chipset from Sonova and is a Made For Any phone device just like the Marvel. That means that it will connect to any cell phone with a Bluetooth radio. So that means, iPhones, Android phones and even dumbphones.

Hands-Free Phone Calls

The hearing aids provide hands-free phone calls from your connected cell phone. You simply press the button on the hearing aid to answer the call and talk away. You can also end the phone call with a simple touch of the button on your hearing aids.

TV Audio Streaming

There is a TV streamer accessory for the device that allows you to stream audio from any TV or sound system directly to your hearing aids without an intermediary streamer. The TV accessory provides excellent sound quality.

Kirkland 9.0 Prices

Overall, the Costco Kirkland Signature 9.0 Hearing Aids seem like pretty good hearing aids considering their purchase price of $1499.99 for a pair. As I said, the technology is not identical to the Phonak Marvel or Unitron Discover line of devices, but they are similar.

Kirkland hearing aids or any of the hearing aids available at Costco do not have any kind of Tinnitus Features inside of their devices, so it's something you need to take into consideration if that's important to you.

Kirkland Signature 9.0 Features

The Kirkland Signature 9.0 uses the Sonova Sword chip for communication, and the features are as follows:

- Third-generation enhanced automatic operating system
- Premium-level classification of environmental sounds and streamed media
- Binaural signal processing and binaural beamforming
- Direct connectivity to any Bluetooth phone with audio streaming to both ears
- Hands-free phone calls with built-in microphones
- 20 fine-tuning channels, 9 automatic programs, 3 manual programs
- Receiver-in-canal (RIC) form factor with 312 battery
- 4 receiver power levels
- Accessories: TV Connector

The Conclusion

The Kirkland 9.0, just like every Kirkland aid before it, is a great offering. It is an ideal hearing aid for people with bog standard, run of the mill hearing loss that responds well to amplification. The absence of a telecoil means that it is not an ideal solution for people who need more than just a hearing aid to get on in complex solutions. As well as that, the lack of a rechargeable option means that Kirkland buyers will miss out on the ease of use of that function.

The Kirkland 9.0 isn't a Phonak Marvel hearing aid, even though it's similar. The Phonak Marvel range offers so much more than the Kirkland, including:

- The call transcription app
- Live real-time remote fine-tuning
- A rechargeable option
- Tinnitus treatment ability
- Access to RogerDirect
- Telecoil options.

That doesn't mean that you should be put off buying them. If you don't think you need those functions, well then the Ks9 is probably an ideal solution for you, who doesn't want the function of the Marvel 90 for an outrageously low fifteen hundred dollars for a pair.

Hearing Aid Types, an introduction

While modern hearing aids have evolved exponentially and they are generally outstanding at what they do. That does not mean that they deliver for every single person. They are just an aid to hearing; they will not replace the natural hearing ability that you have lost.

That warning should not put you off; I give it so that you can manage your expectations. I also provide it so that you can appreciate what you are going to get. My best advice is that you should buy the best set of hearing aids you can afford. I think the key though, is that you buy them from someone who is going to do their level best to help you succeed with them.

Best Advice

Because, if you have a hearing loss, you need to treat it. The growing evidence concerning the consequences of untreated hearing loss is worrying. We see stronger links between untreated hearing loss and cognitive issues. We also see substantial evidence that hearing aids have a beneficial effect on cognitive ability.

We as a population are generally living longer; it appears that treating hearing loss will keep you sharper, more active and generally healthier as you age. There is clear evidence that shows that wearing hearing aids when needed, will contribute to good general health, so what's not to like?

Be realistic with your expectations of the hearing aids that you purchase, the different levels of technology make a big difference to the benefit delivered within different sound environments. I will explain them clearly a little later in the book.

While there is a vast range of hearing aids available, they usually fall within just a few overall general types. Each type has different strengths and weaknesses and differing suitability for different people. Let's explore the different types, including the pros and cons of each one.

What Are The Hearing Aid Types?

Three hearing aid types are most spoken about; they are as follows:

BTE Hearing Aids: These devices are worn with the hearing aid on top of and behind the ear. All of the parts are in the case at the back of the ear, and they are joined to the ear canal with a sound tube and a custom mould or tip.

ITE Hearing Aids: These are custom-made devices, all of the electronics sit in a device that fits in your ear, and they come in many sizes including CIC (Completely in Canal) and IIC (Invisible in Canal).

RIC RITE Hearing Aids: These devices are similar in concept to BTE hearing aids, with the exception that the receiver (the speaker) has been removed from the case that sits at the back of the ear. It is fitted in your ear canal or ear and connected to the case of the hearing aid with a thin wire.

Wireless and Bluetooth Hearing Aids

Before we delve a little deeper into the different types of hearing aids, it is essential to discuss wireless hearing aids and the devices that have become commonly known to the general public as Bluetooth hearing aids. All the hearing device manufacturers have wireless hearing aids, and most have introduced Bluetooth hearing aids over the last few years.

They aren't necessarily the same thing. Let's talk about wireless before I explain Bluetooth later. While wireless hearing aids work with Bluetooth connections, they aren't precisely Bluetooth. Most of the manufacturers designed their own flavour of wireless signal. Wireless communication between hearing aids and between hearing aids and other accessory devices has been a game-changer for people who wear hearing aids.

Not just has it made it easier for people to enjoy their TV, phone calls and group situations, the wireless communication has also enabled jaw-dropping features (at least for us nerds) in the hearing aids that deliver a much better experience for their users.

In the very recent past (since 2017 maybe) many of the hearing aid brands are dropping their own wireless systems and moving towards the direct connection that Bluetooth provides.

RIC Receiver in Canal Hearing Aids

RIC/ RITE hearing aids, sometimes called speaker in the ear, are powerful but discreet hearing aids. Let's take a more in-depth look at them.

RIC / RITE Hearing Aids

DISCREET BEHIND THE EAR DEVICES

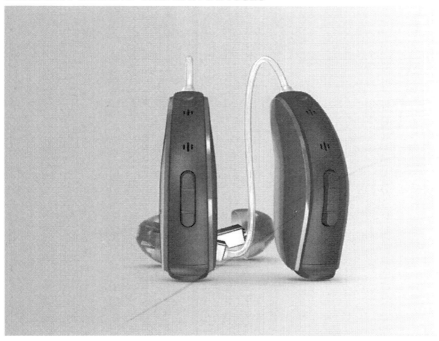

RIC (Receiver in Canal) / RITE (Receiver In The Ear) were first introduced around 2008 as far as I can remember. To produce ever-smaller but more potent Behind The Ear type hearing aids, manufacturers moved the receiver (the speaker part) out of the body of the hearing aid and placed it at the end of a wire that went into the ear canal. Hence, a receiver in canal or receiver in the ear.

The devices have become hugely popular both within the profession and with buyers because they are massively versatile, fitting many types of hearing losses and very discreet. In some cases, they are more discreet than in the ear hearing aids. They do, however, have their pros and cons, let's take a more in-depth look at them.

THE PROS & CONS OF RIC HEARING AIDS

As with many things in life, there are pros and cons with RIC hearing aids; first, let's take a look at the advantages of RIC devices.

What Are The Advantages Of RIC Devices?

Discreet

They are highly discreet devices; although the body of the hearing aid sits behind the ear, they usually are very small and unobtrusive. Unless someone is checking they invariably go unnoticed.

The wire that leads from the body of the hearing aid into the ear canal is tiny and should sit along the crease of your face at the ear. Hence, it is almost unnoticeable as well. Because of these two facts, these are among the most discreet hearing aids available.

Easy Change Receivers

Because the receiver is easily interchangeable, these hearing aids can cover varied hearing losses from mild all the way through to severe to profound. It also means that if the receiver fails, which happens, it is easily changed out for a new one.

That means that the hearing aid does not have to go away for repair for a receiver change, it can be done instantly in the office if the hearing professional has spare receivers. That is a big plus, being without your hearing aid once you are used to wearing it is excruciating.

The pure joy of being able to hear well without massive levels of concentration and straining is only something you appreciate after you have a problem with your hearing aid.

What Are the Disadvantages of RIC Devices

Receiver Issues in RICs/RITEs

The fact that the receiver is placed in the canal or the ear, is both a blessing and a curse. This placement exposes it to the hostile environment that the ear is for electronics. Your ear canal is wet warm and oily, all of the things that electronics tend not to like.

The manufacturers take great pains to protect the receivers with Nano coating materials, enclosed casings and wax guard protectors. However, unless you take good care of the receivers, changing your wax guards when you should, (you probably won't) inevitably wax gets into them.

At best, this can just block the sound outlet; at worst, the wax can ingress into the receiver itself and destroy it. Wax and moisture is the kiss of death for receivers. Thankfully, you're your professional can quickly replace receivers; however, after the manufacturer's warranty is up, you may have to pay for them.

While they vary in cost, they are not expensive; however, if you are replacing them regularly, the cost adds up. I don't want to put you off this device types, they are exceptionally versatile, and I like them. If you are recommended this type of device just be aware of the receiver issues.

Many of the hearing healthcare professionals we partner with can arrange a five-year manufacturer's warranty to cover repairs. Some may charge, some may offer it for free.

If you are considering buying RICs, ask about an extended manufacturer's warranty.

Maybe Too Small!

As I said, RICs / RITEs are tiny and discreet devices, usually the smaller they are, the smaller the battery they use. Both the size of the hearing aid and the size of the battery can cause difficulties for people with dexterity issues. The whole idea of acquiring hearing aids is so that you can wear them and enjoy the genuine benefits of hearing better.

If you have difficulty handling them to put them in, what should be a joy, can quickly turn into a frustrating task at best.

I must say the same about the batteries; small batteries can be a nightmare for people with vision or dexterity issues. Many of the hearing aid manufacturers offer RIC / RITE hearing aids in a variety of sizes and battery sizes, for instance, Phonak offer the Audeo V range in a size 10 battery, a size 312 battery and a size

13 battery. The only caveat is the more substantial the battery, the bigger the hearing aid case.

Contra-indications To Wearing RICs / RITEs

Some people shouldn't wear these type of devices. If you have permanent perforations in your ears or you have had a mastoid operation, these hearing devices aren't really for you.

As you will know if you have these problems, there is an increased risk of middle ear infections and fluid release. Either will destroy the receivers of the hearing aids, because of the nature of your ears with these conditions receiver failures would be an ongoing problem rather than an occasional frustration. We can say the same for people who suffer from wet ears or produce a large amount of earwax; either condition will cause issues for the receivers.

In Finishing

Great devices, they have their pros and cons; proper care will lead to fewer problems.

ITE In The Ear Hearing Aids

In The Ear or custom hearing aids are discreet and popular hearing aids for consumers, let's take a more in-depth look at them.

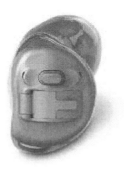

Custom Hearing Aids

ITE, CIC, IIC HEARING AIDS

Custom hearing aids or in the ear hearing aids come in many shapes and sizes, from quite visible Full Shell hearing aids to the so-called hidden hearing aids, the Invisible In Canal or IICs.

Custom hearing aids have been around for a very long time, as I said they come in many shapes and sizes that deliver different levels of power and functionality. They were hugely popular devices, but when the manufacturers introduced RIC / RITE devices, their popularity waned somewhat.

With the introduction of the so-called "Invisible hearing aids" several years ago their popularity has been resurgent. Hearing aid manufacturers are also overcoming some of the technical challenges that reduced the functionality of the minimal custom device types in the recent past.

That has made the devices a better choice for people who need more help in tougher environments but want a very discreet package. Many of the manufacturers now offer small wireless-enabled completely in canal devices, which eliminates the traditional trade-off between discretion and functionality. Let's talk about the types.

Invisible Hearing Aids

Invisible hearing aids or hidden hearing aids have been with us for a while; however, initially, they weren't that hidden. That has changed dramatically. The manufacturers cracked the difficulties that precluded them from making truly invisible hearing aids.

Since then every manufacturer has introduced invisible in the canal hearing aid ranges. They fit deeply in the ear canal, and you cannot see the faceplate easily. They are genuinely discreet hearing devices and have been well received. There are, of course, disadvantages, the IIC hearing aids are often too small to be wireless.

However, in the recent past, some of the manufacturers, Starkey, Siemens and Oticon in particular, have delivered wireless IIC devices, that's wireless, not Bluetooth enabled.

For some, the trade-off between discretion and wireless functionality is an easy choice. They forgo wireless capability for the discretion; however, I believe there is a lot to be said for wireless capability. I think wireless accessories are outstanding solutions and used well they have changed the lives of hard of hearing people dramatically for the better.

But hey, that's just me. Invisible hearing aids are not suitable for everyone for several reasons; some reasons I will discuss later when talking about the overall pros and cons of custom hearing aids. However, there is one that is particular to invisible hearing aids, canal size and shape. If your canal is not the right shape or size, you are out of luck. Let's answer a few questions about invisible hearing aids

What are invisible hearing aids?
Invisible hearing aids are deep fitting custom made hearing devices that sit deep within the ear canal. More often than not, you can't see the faceplate of the hearing aid. For this reason, they have been given the name invisible. The first manufacturer to introduce modern invisible hearing aids was Starkey, they introduced the SoundLens, and it began the race across all hearing device manufacturers to add their version. Every manufacturer has now launched a hidden hearing aid option.

These hearing instrument types are called by different names by the various manufacturers, sound lens, Nano, IIC invisible in the canal or just plain invisible hearing aids. No matter the official title, they all amount to pretty much the same thing, deep canal hearing aids.

The battleground has now extended as some of the device manufacturers have now introduced wireless invisible hearing devices. Something which up to now has been technically challenging. We would expect more of the hearing brands to begin offering wireless invisible instruments over the next year. Although this market is small, while you might expect everyone to want one, not everyone is suitable.

Are invisible hearing devices suitable for everyone?
The short answer is no, not at this time, while your hearing loss obviously needs to be taken into account, the major stumbling block to suitability is usually the size and shape of your ear canal. If your ear canal is either too small, too narrow or too awkward, you won't be suitable for these devices; It is as simple as that.

Even with advancements in technology, that will probably remain the case for a few years to come. The manufacturers simply need a finite amount of space to fit all of the components in, if your canal does not offer that space, you are out of luck.

Are invisible hearing aids available on the NHS?
That is a question that we get a lot; unfortunately, the answer is no. However, there is exceptionally discreet receiver in canal hearing aids available on the NHS.

How much do invisible hearing aids cost?
Generally, they are no more expensive than a different hearing aid type from the same technology level. In other words, you

typically don't pay a premium for an invisible hearing aid. I say generally, because there always may be exceptions. For instance, the Phonak Virto B Titanium (which comes in an invisible version) is slightly more expensive than a similar traditional Virto B hearing aid at the minute.

Invisible hearing aids with Bluetooth?

Again, we get asked this quite a bit; the answer is yes but no, hahaha, let me explain. There are wireless invisible hearing aids, but no, they don't run on the Bluetooth connection. In the recent past, some of the hearing aid brands have released wireless invisible hearing aids.

They are wirelessly equipped, and they will connect to the manufacturer's audio streaming devices. I think this is a fantastic move forward because I believe wireless hearing aids were a tremendous innovation. There are no Made For iPhone invisible hearing aids; there are no direct connection devices available right now.

What type of hearing loss will invisible hearing aids work with?

Generally, invisible hearing aids are suitable for moderate flattish type hearing losses. Those are usually the best types of hearing losses served by the devices. Let's take a look at other hearing loss types.

High-Frequency hearing loss and invisible hearing aids

Generally, invisible hearing aids aren't suitable for people with high-frequency hearing loss. The problem is that they have a good low-frequency hearing, so putting a device into the ear canal causes intolerable occlusion. That can be by-passed by ensuring the invisible hearing aid fits into the bony part of the ear canal. In theory, this should stop any occlusion, however, getting the device that deep in the canal can be difficult, and it may be uncomfortable.

Moderate hearing loss and IIC

As I said, invisible hearing devices are ideal for flattish moderate hearing loss, there are no difficulties with occlusion, and the hearing aid output is perfect for this type of loss.

Severe Hearing Loss and hidden hearing aids

In general, most hearing aid professionals would not offer invisible hearing aids to someone with a severe hearing loss. They are not ideal because they don't provide much headroom, which simply means if the hearing loss gets much worse, the hearing aid is useless. However, there are invisible hearing aids suitable for severe hearing loss from Signia.

Profound hearing loss, and Invisible In Canal

There are no invisible hearing aids that are currently suitable for someone who suffers from a profound hearing loss.

The pros and cons of invisible hearing instruments

They are similar to most custom hearing aids; the positioning of them may well be optimal for hearing devices. That position deep in the canal allows the outer ear and ear canal to do its job, funnel sound naturally towards the eardrum. That is probably the most significant benefit of these types of devices. However, that positioning means all of the electronics are open to wax and moisture in the ear canal. That means that they need a lot of care and attention from the user. They also need dehumidifying regularly.

If you are prepared to take care of these hearing aids well, then I would say go ahead with them. However, you will need to take care of them to avoid electronics failures. As I said, while there are wireless invisible hearing aids, generally speaking, most invisible hearing aids are non-wireless enabled.

Completely In Canal Hearing Aids / Mini In Canal

Completely in canal or CIC hearing aids are pretty discreet devices that will go unnoticed except by the keenest eye. Up to recently, they were predominantly non-wireless; however, in just the recent past, many manufacturers have released wireless-enabled CICs.

I think that this is a fantastic breakthrough; however, wireless-enabled devices are slightly bigger than non-wireless CICs, so you need to consider that before you go ahead if complete discretion is your objective. What is hugely interesting is that some manufacturers have managed to fit directional microphones on CICs, this again is a recent breakthrough.

Directional microphones give real assistance in noisy environments. However, this is the first time they have been on CICs, so it will be interesting to see the effect they have. Early reports indicate that they deliver better speech clarity in the group and noisy situations.

Again though, directional mics make the CIC slightly more substantial, I believe though, that like wireless, the functionality is well worth the trade-off. Mini in canal hearing aids are all of the above with the exception that they are slightly larger, most mini in canals would come with wireless functionality and directional microphones.

Full Shell & Half Shell Hearing Aids

They are as they sound, larger custom hearing aids that sit in the concha or bowl of the ear. The half-shell fills half the concha, and the full shell fills the whole concha. The traditional benefit of these devices has been more features, more power and physical controls like programme button and volume controls.

Recently, with the introduction of wireless capability and more powerful CIC solutions, those benefits have all but become negated. However, these devices still have advantages; they usually have bigger battery sizes, which allow them to work longer between changes and they are easier to handle for people with dexterity and vision problems.

THE PROS & CONS OF CUSTOM HEARING AIDS

Yes, you guessed it, there are most definitely advantages and disadvantages to custom hearing aids. Let's take a more in-depth look at what they are.

What Are The Advantages Of Custom Hearing Devices?

Discreet

The smaller devices are highly discreet, and the invisible hearing aids are, in fact, invisible. The larger devices are of course not as discreet.

Easy To Handle

Because the devices are all in one unit, they can be easy to handle and to place in the ear, especially the larger hearing aids.

What Are The Disadvantages of Custom Hearing Devices?

Receiver Issues, Microphone Issues

Like RIC / RITE devices, the receiver is placed in the ear canal. However, it is better protected than the receivers in RICs. Again this placement exposes not just the receiver but all of the electronic components including the microphones to the hostile environment of the ear.

The manufacturers take great pains to protect both the receivers and the microphones. However, unless you take good care of your hearing aids, changing your wax guards when you should and cleaning the microphones, you are looking at possible failures.

Dirt and Wax, a Nightmare for Hearing Aids

At best, wax or dirt can just block the sound outlet or microphone inlet; at worst, it can make its way into the components itself and destroy them. As we said, wax and moisture is the kiss of death for electronics. The manufacturers have done an excellent job of protecting those sensitive components in most cases.

It is rare for anything other than the microphone or receiver to fail; chipset failures are that rare that they are remarked upon with surprise.

In the case of custom hearing aids, if there is a failure, they will have to be sent off for repair, which can take a varying amount of time. If the fault is under warranty, it will be repaired free of charge; if not, you will have to pay a fee. If you are having them repaired regularly, the cost adds up.

Good Clean and Care

The key to success with these hearing aid types is an excellent clean and care routine that involves drying. The better you take care of these hearing aids, the better they will perform. Again, I don't want to put you off this device types, they are fantastic devices, and I like them. If you are recommended this type of device just be aware of the inherent issues.

As we said, many of the hearing healthcare professionals we partner with can arrange a five-year manufacturer's warranty to cover repairs. Some may charge, some may offer it for free. If you are considering buying custom hearing aids, ask about an extended manufacturer's warranty.

Maybe Too Small!

Some of the custom hearing aids are tiny and discreet devices, as with RIC / RITE devices, the smaller the device, the smaller the battery they use. With the smaller custom devices, the size of the hearing aid and the size of the battery can cause difficulties for people with dexterity issues.

If you have trouble handling the hearing aids or putting the batteries in, what should be a joy can quickly turn into a frustrating task. The larger custom devices are easier to handle and use larger batteries that are easier to handle.

Contra-indications To Wearing Custom Hearing Aids

As with RICs and RITE devices, some people shouldn't wear these type of devices. It is pretty much the same as RICs if you have permanent perforations in your ears or you have had a mastoid operation these hearing devices aren't really for you.

The same can be said for people who suffer from wet ears or produce a large amount of earwax; either condition will cause issues for the hearing aids. Even though they have significantly increased the power output in this type of hearing aids, they still might not be suitable for your hearing loss.

If they aren't, don't let vanity win, get a hearing aid that is suitable for your hearing loss. That will translate into better hearing, which will help you lead a better life.

In Finishing

Again these are great devices. Generally, they are quite reliable, but they do need care and attention to ensure they keep on keeping on.

BTE Behind The Ear Hearing Aids

We love BTE hearing aids, probably the most reliable hearing devices you can buy.

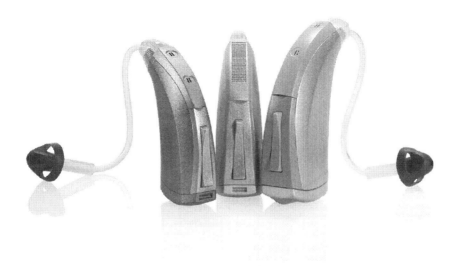

BTE HEARING AIDS

Behind The Ear or BTE hearing aids have been around for a very long time. In the recent past, they have got smaller, more versatile and more powerful. Behind the ear hearing aids are self-contained units with all of the components in the case. Over recent years they have gotten much smaller than they once were. They are hugely versatile devices, and they will fit nearly every hearing loss.

Usually, the manufacturers will make different styles for differing losses, one for most losses from mild to severe and one often labelled a superpower for profound hearing loss. Even the superpower devices have become quite small in comparison to the older styles. The hearing aid is connected to the ear through a coupling, in some cases, it is via a tube and ear mould, in the case of the hearing aids to the left it is with a thin tube and instant fit tip. The actual fittings are varied and usually based on hearing loss.

THE PROS & CONS OF BTE HEARING AIDS

We are finding it hard to think of disadvantages really, but we will give it the old college try. Let's take a look at what you can expect from BTE devices.

What Are The Advantages Of BTE Hearing Devices

Fully Functional Hearing Solutions

BTE hearing aids nearly always have a full load of hardware including volume controls, programme buttons and telecoils. The telecoil is a useful addition if you want access to loop systems in public buildings like churches, conference centres, and the post office.

Many taxis in London are fitted with loop systems. Even though wireless communication systems in hearing aids are now the norm, the telecoil is still a good thing to have. The only issues that occur concerning it are how well the loop system is working or how well it has been fitted. This can affect audio quality.

Extremely Reliable Hearing Aids

BTE hearing aids are probably the most reliable of hearing aids; they very seldom fail. Because all of the components are encased in the hearing aid and the hearing aid is worn at the back of the ear, very little or no wax or moisture can get at them.

When something goes wrong with a BTE, it tends to be either the physical controls or the microphones. Nearly all of the manufacturers have introduced new types of microphone covers that almost completely enclose the microphones. So even microphone failure may be a thing of the past.

Easy To Use

BTE hearing aids tend to be easy to handle and place in the ear, so for people with dexterity or vision issues; they are a good choice.

What Are The Disadvantages of BTE Hearing Devices

Haven't a Clue

We are wracking our brains here and really can't think of anything, maybe discretion? Even that isn't true, a small BTE with a thin tube is a very discreet hearing aid to wear. It would be almost as discreet as many of the RIC / RITE devices. Okay, the larger BTEs are not the most discreet, but I would always go for long-term reliability every time. A hearing aid is of no use to you if it is broke and BTEs very rarely break.

Some people complain about BTEs and glasses; they get in the way of each other. I think that is probably a function of physiology. It depends on how much your ears stick out or don't.

Contra-indications To Wearing BTEs

Sorry, again we are stuck for any here. Perhaps if you have tiny ears?

Bluetooth / Made For iPhone Hearing Aids

Bluetooth hearing aids (Made For iPhone hearing aids are Bluetooth hearing aids) are direct connection devices. By that I mean they use some sort of onboard Bluetooth radio to connect directly to another device without the assistance of an intermediary streamer.

The device that they connect to can be an assistive listening device designed by the hearing aid manufacturer or an iPhone. The original LiNX from GN Resound was the very first Bluetooth hearing device to come onto the market. The category is generally known as Made For iPhone or direct connection hearing aids.

The designed the LiNX to also connect to GN Resound's Unite wireless accessories, which were designed to connect to phones, audio systems and TVs. What made them different from everything else at the time was that they could connect directly to an iPhone without any intermediary device. They were the very first to have this ability although they were followed quickly by the Halo from Starkey.

At the time of writing, every major hearing aid brand has released devices that will connect directly to iPhones without intermediary streamers. Many of the brands, such as Oticon and Signia, have released complete ranges of direct connection devices. That appears to be the way most of the brands are going.

The Problem with Bluetooth

All these hearing aids are pretty outstanding devices and the fact that they connect directly without an add-on is celebrated by many users. However, they have their issues. Generally, those issues are caused by Bluetooth. Although Bluetooth technology has gotten better, it is still a finicky technology which occasionally just does its own thing.

Like dropping the connection for no reason and then refusing to find the device it was just connected to. Believe me, I use Bluetooth every day for information transfer purposes, and it can be infuriating. It often works exceptionally well for weeks at a time and then it doesn't, for no apparent reason.

Unfortunately, the hearing aid manufacturers can't control this; it is just a function of Bluetooth. Again, I wouldn't let this hold you back, just be aware of the problem when you are making a decision.

Made For Any Phone Hearing Aids

In the recent past, Sonova (owns Phonak, Unitron) has introduced Made For Any phone hearing aids. These devices use the traditional Bluetooth headset protocol to connect to any mobile phone with a Bluetooth radio. They will pretty much connect to any device with a Bluetooth radio, including computers or even TVs.

Hands-Free Calls

The Sonova range of devices is the only hearing aids to provide hands-free calls. When your phone rings, you simply press a button on your hearing aid and chat away. No need to touch your phone.

Stereo Streaming

The Sonova devices also offer stereo streaming of media from your phone or connected device.

Power Hungry

The system is power hungry though, Sonova says that they have managed to reduce the battery drain to something akin to a typical Made For iPhone hearing aid. If you are buying these devices, go rechargeable or be prepared to change your batteries every couple of days.

Made For Android

Made For Android is now a reality with the introduction of Android 10. At present, there are only two hearing aid ranges that use the system. Starkey Livio and Resound LiNX Quattro ranges will connect to certain Android-powered phones. The key here is that the phone needs to be running Android 10, and it needs the right hardware.

When ASHA (the connection protocol for Android) was introduced I expected all of the manufacturers to quickly adopt it. That hasn't happened, it may well be because of the introduction of a completely new Bluetooth standard for hearing aids.

That standard will probably be released late in 2020 and it should ensure that hearing aids can connect to any Bluetooth device that uses it. Perhaps, they are all waiting on that instead?

Rechargeable Hearing Aids

Rechargeable hearing aids have been with us for a while; both Siemens and Hansaton have provided rechargeable hearing aids for many years. Up to recently, they have not been hugely popular. That has changed dramatically, let me first tell you why they weren't popular and then explain what will change that forever.

The main issue with the first rechargeable hearing aids was battery technology. The batteries simply could not be trusted to power modern hearing aids and the demands of streaming audio for a full day without interruption.

Not just that, the life of rechargeable batteries tended to be about a year. After that, they did not continue to hold their charge well and needed to be replaced. For most hearing aid providers, it made little sense to recommend them to prospective users. They were perceived to be a novelty and never gained traction.

What's Changed?

The battery technology has dramatically evolved, Phonak, quickly followed by Signia, introduced the first-ever rechargeable hearing aids powered by Lithium-ion batteries. Lithium-ion as a power source is more capable and a far better option for hearing aid use.

The Lithium-ion technology delivers a full 24 hours of use on a single three-hour charge. The use time changes when you include streaming audio time, so if you use your hearing aids like wireless headphones for music, TV or phone connection, you should still get 16 hours of use.

Lithium-ion is also capable of far more charge-recharge cycles. However, initially, there was some worry that the power pack might only offer peak performance for three to four years, which meant that the power pack would need to be changed during the lifetime of the hearing aids. That worry has receded somewhat because several of the brands have undertaken accelerated cycle testing that appears to show the power packs will deliver up to six years before changing them needs to be considered.

Initially, only two brands introduced Lithium-Ion powered rechargeable hearing aids. The rest of the brands introduced Silver-Zinc powered rechargeable hearing aids powered by the Z-Power system. That has changed though; nearly every brand has now changed to lithium-ion as a power source. Silver Zinc batteries have fallen out of favour.

Why does this change everything?

Probably most importantly, consumers want it; they want it badly. If you are an experienced user you will probably know what I mean, if you aren't, let me explain. Most experienced users have a giant size pain in their arse (Irish technical term) with disposable hearing aid batteries. They are fiddly, easy to drop and generally irritating, not just that they are also an ongoing cost.

Generally, the cost is negligible; however, they are still an ongoing cost that many users resent. There is also the whole hassle of making sure you have spare batteries wherever you go.

Sounds easy right? Nahhhhh, as most people will tell you, the day they forgot to pack their extra batteries was the day the hearing aids run out unexpectedly.

So, we have a congruence of two states of being, Hearing aid providers are more likely to recommend rechargeable hearing aids and the market, in general, will be exceptionally receptive to them.

Why Should You Consider Rechargeable Hearing Aids?

There are many reasons why you should consider buying rechargeable hearing aids, and I would like to set them out here. Generally, rechargeable hearing aid options are no more, or little more expensive than the models that use traditional hearing aid batteries, so the cost of adoption is negligible.

Ease of Use

Rechargeable hearing aids offer real ease of use to you, no fiddling around with little batteries every few days. The size of hearing aid batteries, and hearing aids themselves, can be irritating and troubling to users, especially if they have eyesight or dexterity issues.

Just removing the disposable battery from the packaging can be a mini nightmare for some people, let alone opening the battery compartment and getting the damn battery in there! So, if you have decreased dexterity or a condition that numb the fingertips, such as arthritis, diabetic neuropathy, and Parkinson's disease.

Well then, rechargeable hearing aids are most definitely for you. You simply put rechargeable hearing aids into the charger at night, and in the morning, they are ready for use. More than that, you don't need to remember to buy batteries, you don't need to remember to carry spares, you never run out and generally your battery won't let you down at the very worst moment.

Good for The World

Rechargeable batteries are far greener and better for the environment than disposable hearing aid batteries. During a five year period, you will need, on average, 520 disposable batteries.

You will need to replace the lithium-ion powerpack after six years. The thing is though; you might be in the market for new hearing aids after six years. So, you may never replace it. They will still have enough life to act as your spare pair when needed.

Cost-Neutral

The lithium-ion power packs will probably cost the price of a standard repair. That varies from place to place, but in Ireland, it is around €180. So, for two, it will be €360. Six years of traditional at the very best price of €50 a year is close to that, really close.

So, the cost is probably relatively neutral. For those people who don't shop for their hearing aid batteries online, rechargeable batteries are probably a far cheaper option.

All types of hearing aids?

At present, this new renaissance of rechargeable is mostly available in BTE and RIC models. While Starkey has introduced a rechargeable custom, making custom hearing aids rechargeable is a complex operation. Generally speaking, it would not be difficult to make a large custom hearing aid rechargeable (such as a full shell ITE). However, making a small ITE like a CIC rechargeable is complex.

We also have no idea about the long-term reliability of the devices. So I think it will be a while before we see other manufacturers introduce them. With the advent of the COVID-19, that time-line may even be longer.

Phonak Rechargeable

Phonak kick-started this new movement with the introduction of their Audeo B-R or Belong-Rechargeable. The device is a Receiver in Canal device, and it is available in their top three levels of technology. Interestingly they didn't offer it in their lowest entry-level range. The device can handle several levels of receiver, so it covers hearing losses from mild to profound.

They say that no matter the level of the receiver, the device will last for twenty-four hours between charges with up to eighty minutes streaming of audio wirelessly. That is pretty impressive. They have found in field trials that the devices will last for up to fifteen hours with five hours of streaming, which is pretty much a full day for most users. That would mean that you would get quite a bit of answering your mobile and watching the television in as well.

The devices will run for six hours after a thirty-minute charge, and a full charge takes three hours in total. They quickly followed up with the introduction of their Bolero B P-R, which is a BTE powered by the same rechargeable power pack. They offer the same stats for it.

Audeo Marvel
The new Audeo Marvel range from Phonak offers two rechargeable Receiver In Canal hearing aids. One without a telecoil, which is available right now, and one without a telecoil, which will be available late 2019.

The Marvel rechargeables are available in every level of Phonak technology, and because the initial ones are RICs, they will cover every hearing loss from mild to severe to profound.

Signia Rechargeable Hearing Aids
Signia quickly joined the fray with the introduction of their Cellion Primax devices. Again, these are Receiver in Canal devices, and again, they can take many levels of receivers. Signia introduced the Cellion in all its levels of technology. They say that the Cellion devices will last 24 hours with limitless streaming. That is exceptionally impressive if it proves true (no reason to doubt them!)

Signia Nx range
Signia quickly followed up the Cellion with the introduction of a variety of rechargeable hearing aids on the Nx platform. They now offer three rechargeable RICs, the Pure Charge N Go, the Styletto and the Styletto Connect, and a rechargeable BTE, the Motion Charge N Go.

Signia say that you will be able to stream up to five hours per day and still benefit from 17 hours of battery life before needing to recharge with the Motion and Pure. The Styletto Connect devices will deliver 16 hours of use with five hours of streaming. That's pretty good streaming time and battery life. The Styletto is a non-Bluetooth enabled aid and will deliver a full day of use on one charge.

Oticon Rechargeable Digital Hearing Aids

Oticon was a little late to the party with their Rechargeable hearing aids offer. Oticon originally went down the route of the Z Power Silver Zinc technology with their Opn range. However, they had quite a few problems with the silver-zinc systems, and they have now introduced a lithium-ion powered hearing aid on the Opn S range.

Resound Rechargeable Digital Hearing Aids

Resound introduced their rechargeable hearing aids in August 2017. They initially went down the route of using the Z Power Silver-Zinc battery technology. Like Oticon, they have now gone to lithium-ion powered devices in their new Quattro range.

Starkey Rechargeable Digital Hearing Aids

Starkey also initially went for Z Power for their rechargeable hearing aids. They have also now introduced lithium-ion powered rechargeable hearing aids.

Unitron Rechargeable Digital Hearing Aids

Unitron quickly followed their stablemate Phonak (both owned by Sonova) with their own rechargeable hearing aids. However, unlike Phonak, they went for the Z Powered Silver-Zinc option. They first introduced a Receiver In Canal rechargeable option but have since followed with a Behind The Ear Option. With the launch of their new Discovery platform, they have gone with lithium-ion.

Widex Rechargeable Digital Hearing Aids

Widex were practically the last to the party with rechargeable hearing aids. They have been working on Fuel Cell technology for many years, and it will change the powering of hearing aids forever.

I say without hesitation that fuel cell technology is a paradigm shift, and I expected to see it introduced in 2019. Unfortunately, it wasn't to be. Fuel cell tech is now dead for the moment. Widex have now announced the introduction of a lithium-ion powered rechargeable hearing aid with the launch of the Moment.

What Are The Pros and Cons of Rechargeable Hearing Aids?

Some people have warned people off rechargeable hearing aids for different reasons, I think they are exceptionally beneficial, but there are pros and cons, let's talk about the types and what they have to offer.

Lithium-ion Rechargeable hearing aids

Most of the hearing aid brands now offer Lithium-ion rechargeable hearing aids. In the case of Phonak, the power pack is a sealed, integrated system. Signia have delivered something similar, but different. The systems offer pros for safety and cons for the use case. Let me explain, Lithium-ion can be a fire risk if the battery is damaged, sealing the battery in the body of the hearing aid means that it is protected from mishandling.

However, sealing it in the case also means that the user cannot replace it. Lithium-ion can be expected to deliver for between four and five years, so that means the battery pack will have to be replaced after four or five years because it will not be providing what it should.

The hearing aids will have to be sent back to the factory, and it will also have a cost attached. From what I know, Phonak at least has said that they will replace battery packs in the future as a standard repair, which means it won't be a ridiculous cost.

As I said, Signia has done it differently; their power pack is a sealed unit. However, they have designed the outer case to ensure that the power pack can be replaced in the office as opposed to the factory.

The Cons of Lithium-Ion Rechargeable Hearing Aids

- **Safety**: Lithium-ion is a poison, and hearing aids are small enough to swallow, presenting a hazard to children and pets. Lithium-ion has the potential to go on fire if damaged badly enough.

- **Sealed Case**: The fire hazard of the tech dictates that the lithium-ion battery is integrated into a sealed case. If it runs out of power while still in use, the hearing aid cannot run on a standard disposable battery but must be taken out of commission while it recharges. And when a lithium-ion battery reaches the end of its life, it can't be replaced by the user but must be swapped out by the manufacturer (Phonak devices) or the professional (Signia Devices).

- **Power Limitations**: If you stream a lot of audio (from an MP3 player or mobile phone, etc.), there's a possibility the batteries may not last the full 24-hour day. In fact, Phonak seem to think that if you stream up to about five hours, the aids will last 14 to 16 hours. This shouldn't affect most people, though since 12-16 hours would be a typical day of hearing aid use.

- **Larger Footprint:** The footprint of Lithium-Ion is bigger than the other option, which means bigger hearing aids.

The Pros of Lithium-Ion Rechargeable Hearing Aids

- **No more fiddly battery changes:** The technology ensures that you no longer have to worry about the expense of disposable hearing aid batteries, nor do you have to worry about changing them.

- **24 hours of continuous use:** The technology has finally reached the one-charge-per-day standard. You should be able to get up to 24 hours use with up to **5 hours streaming.**

- **Easy charging**: Simply drop it in your charger, no hassle.

Hearing Aid Technology Levels

Hearing aid technology levels can be confusing at best, why is one better than the other? Here is what you need to know.

LET'S TALK HEARING AID TECHNOLOGY

Once upon a time, there were three hearing aid technology levels, which were known in the profession as low end, mid-range and high end. Then most of the hearing aid manufacturers introduced four, loosely they are called, basic, standard, advanced and premium and that is the designations I will use here for clarity.

The Life of a Hearing Aid

We hear many times that a hearing aid has a life of about five years, that isn't quite true. What is meant by that is, hearing aid technology moves forward every five years. Hearing aids themselves can last for over a decade with care and attention.

So if you buy one today, you may still be wearing it in ten or twelve years, the available hearing aid technology will have changed dramatically twice in that time. Doesn't mean that there is anything wrong with your hearing aid, it just means that there are things that are radically better available.

Let's take a look at those levels and what you can expect from them in general. Every couple of years a hearing aid manufacturer releases a new product range, once it was every four years, but it seems to have accelerated to almost every two years in the recent past.

For clarity purposes, a product range may be referred to as a chipset, a platform or a family by differing people within the profession. Each new product range will have four levels of technology.

We said that there used to be three technology levels in hearing aids, but that had changed, we kind of feel what the manufacturers have done in most cases is split the mid-range into two levels. They are a lower mid-range, which is what we are calling standard, and a higher mid-range, which is what we are calling advanced.

Usually, within each technology level, there will be every hearing aid type that they produce. For instance, Widex has introduced its new product range the Moment, the Moment product range is based on the new Moment chipset, and it has four levels of technology, the 440 which is top of the range or premium technology, the 330, the 220 and the 110 which is the basic level of technology.

Each of those Widex technology levels will have a full family of hearing aids, including custom, RICS and soon, BTEs. Nearly every manufacturer offers hearing aid products in this manner, some use different names to mark different technology levels, but most use some sort of name and numeral combination. Phonak like to confuse everyone by giving their hearing aid types different names, but at least they stick to the numeral using the number 90 for their premium top of the range devices, 70, 50 and finally 30 for their basic level.

How Hearing Aids Work

Before we launch into the different levels of technology, let's talk quickly about what hearing aids are. Hearing aids have changed dramatically over the last few decades with the advent of digital technology. At their core, hearing aids have always been made of the same four basic parts: a microphone, a processor, a receiver (the speaker), and a power source (the battery).

In simple terms, the microphone picks up the sounds and passes it to the processor. The processor enhances the signal following its programming and delivers it to the receiver, which provides the amplified signal to the ear canal.

The power source delivers the power needed to make the magic happen. The introduction of digital technology transformed hearing aids allowing manufacturers to introduce ever more powerful processors in smaller packages. In modern hearing aids, the signal picked up by the microphone is converted from analogue to digital before being processed; this allows for a much deeper manipulation and enhancement of the sound.

This manipulation is how noise reduction and other hearing aid features work. The signal is then converted back from digital to analogue before the receiver delivers the enhanced signal into the ear canal. It is nearly impossible to get an analogue hearing aid now, virtually all of the hearing aids manufactured in the world are now digital. Okay, let's take a look at what the tech levels are and more importantly, what they can do for you.

Basic technology hearing aids

Each manufacturer has a basic level of technology, they may not call it exactly that, but for clarity that is the label, it is getting. This level of technology is designed to work for people who are relatively sedentary (don't get out much).

As I have said, this might be the basic level, but it will still be on the latest chipset available from the manufacturer. Basic level hearing aids are usually just that, quite basic, they will have features such as directional microphones and maybe even some noise reduction, more on both later, but generally they will be basic, and they will be manually controlled.

However, that is beginning to change, Phonak has just introduced its latest Venture platform and the basic hearing aid technology the V30 is an automatic hearing aid. It is limited to only two sound situations, but that is an exciting development none the less.

Other manufacturers will follow suit in their next generation of hearing aids. It is just like an arms race when one does it; the others have to follow suit.

Lifestyle help from basic hearing aid technology

You can expect basic technology to help you in less complex sound situations. That means that you can expect to hear well in one to one conversations, even if the person is talking to you from another room (within reason, if you own a thirty bedroom mansion, all bets are off). You can also expect them to help you with small groups, family around the kitchen table, for instance.

They should also help you with TV and Radio, although both can be a little difficult because of the quality of audio from different stations. Depending on the car you drive, this level of technology should also help you with understanding conversation in the car.

Well programmed basic hearing aids will help you somewhat with limited noise if you take the time to learn coping strategies like turning your back to the noise and seating yourself in a way that minimises exposure to it. However, once the noise level rises, they will begin to let you down.

That is where our love of wireless accessories comes in, if you use a remote microphone accessory with a basic level of hearing aids, it will help you in noise. It will give you that extra bit of help you need to hear your companion; it will also open up other opportunities to hear better in different situations.

In the car, you simply hand the remote mic to your passenger, and you will be able to hear them quite clearly. Having issues with the TV? Put your remote mic down by the speaker, or use the cable that comes with it to plug into the audio out of the TV. By no means is it a replacement for higher technology hearing aids, but when you are working on a budget, it can give you the extra edge you need.

Standard technology hearing aids

Again, each manufacturer has a standard level of technology, which is second from the bottom. These devices are aimed at people who are a little more active. The features in these hearing aids will be slightly better than the basic features and are designed to help you hear in somewhat more challenging sound situations.

This level of technology is designed for someone more active in their life. This level of technology has dramatically improved over the years, to give you an idea, the current hearing aids at this level would easily be as good as flagship models from five years ago.

Lifestyle help from standard hearing aid technology

You can expect all of the support that a basic hearing aid would deliver but better, and on top of that, you can expect assistance in group situations, small meetings, out and about at the shops and in restaurants.

Again, this is based on the noise levels present; this level isn't going to help you to hear well in a boisterous restaurant on a Saturday night, think moderate levels of background noise in most situations.

Again, wireless hearing aid accessories can make up for any difficulties in different situations, and you should also consider them. We believe they are worth the extra expense in most cases.

Advanced technology hearing aids

This level of technology is ideal for active people delivering excellent sound quality and speech clarity in most situations they will find themselves in. This level of technology has dramatically improved in the last few years; it seems that most of the manufacturers are keeping a lot of their top-end technology features in the advanced ranges.

They are dumbing them down slightly, but not much, it has been interesting to watch, especially over the last year. For instance, the Widex 330 is almost as good as the 440 range, and the Phonak V70 is nearly as good as the V90 range. There are clear differences between them, and there are valid reasons why you would choose higher-end technology, but they are close nonetheless.

The main differences between this level and the next up are the binaural processing of hearing aid features. Put simply; hearing aids work exceptionally well when they make decisions as a pair, that extends to the functions involved in delivering better hearing.

In the flagship models from brands, the features work in a combined and consolidated manner using the communication between hearing aids.

That really does deliver the best and most natural sound and clarity. Advanced technology level hearing aids may have most of the top-end features, but they don't work together in that combined way. Nevertheless, they are exceptional hearing aids generally.

Lifestyle help from advanced hearing aid technology

Again, you can expect all of the support you get from the two previous levels of hearing technology but better. Advanced hearing aid technology can be expected to assist you in even complex sound situations, especially if you use coping strategies well.

Usually, at this level, you can expect real help with hearing better in situations like large auditoriums, open plan buildings like churches. You should be able to hear quite well at the theatre; music should be a far better experience.

In general, speech clarity in noisier situations should be pretty good. So if you are an active individual who likes to socialise, goes to some meetings and gets out and about to social events, these may well be the hearing aids for you.

We know we are boring you with our obsession with wireless accessories, but hey good honest advice remember? Yes, wireless accessories that are chosen with the situations you really want to hear in mind will help you even more.

Premium level hearing aids

This level of technology is where hearing aid manufacturers deliver all of their very latest features. This level of technology is for people who simply have to hear well in almost every situation. They are designed to handle the most complex sound situations and deliver the best speech clarity and most natural sound.

In this level, the hearing aids will genuinely work as a pair, deciding on how the sound is processed to deliver the very best hearing possible. The decision-making process and the application of the hearing aid features are undertaken in a binaural manner, and because it uses the power of two separate processors, these are always the most powerful hearing aids available (in computing power).

Lifestyle help from premium hearing aids

Pretty much what you would expect, everything that the rest can do but exceptionally better. Premium hearing aid technology is designed to deliver the very best possible hearing and speech clarity in even complex sound situations.

These type of devices are designed for active people who need to hear well everywhere. Remember, though; you will not be delivered super hearing even at this level of technology you will, they design hearing aids to give you the best experience with your residual level of hearing.

They are not designed to, nor can they give you back your normal hearing or better than normal hearing. Oh, and yes, wireless accessories are still an option worth thinking about even at this level.

Hearing Aid Features

Let's Talk Hearing Aid Features

Technology levels and hearing aid features are linked, the better the technology level, the better the feature that is used. The feature set of any hearing aid is dependent on the level of technology of the hearing aid and the manufacturer.

The flagship or highest technology hearing aids from each manufacturer have the best feature set available from them. First of all, when we speak about features in the profession, we are usually not talking about physical features but hearing aid algorithms or mini programmes that run on the processor.

The easiest way to understand is to compare it to a smartphone; a smartphone runs on an overall system like Google's Android or Apple's IOS, however, within that system, there are apps available to you that do different jobs.

Hearing aids and their features are not unlike that concept. Many people get a little snowed under when they try to understand features, and we can understand that. Modern digital hearing aids have a ridiculous amount of different features designed to deliver different levels of benefit to hearing aid users.

All modern hearing aids will have some mixture of different level of features, so we are going to try and investigate them and tell you in plain language what they do. Please forgive me in advance, I am a nerd, and this stuff excites me.

What are the real-world benefits of hearing aid features?

As I discuss the hearing aid features, I will try and translate them into real-world benefits for you. Just explaining what they are and what they do is simply not enough. So without further blah, let's have a look.

Audible indicators in hearing aids

Right at the basics, an audible indicator informs you of some sort of change in the hearing aids you are wearing. For instance, if you change the programme, or if the volume control has changed or that your battery is running low.

In most hearing aids, these tones are usually a beep or melody type sound. Widex are one of the only manufacturers that employ real speech to announce the programme that you are on and whether your battery is low.

They have even made this feature available in many world languages. That is a clear indication of why Widex is a little different to everyone else; they think clearly about the little details that would help.

They are one of the very few manufacturers to use this feature, and it is available across their range of hearing aids no matter what the technology level.

What are the advantages for you?

Audible indicators allow you to know what is happening in your hearing aids at any one time, for instance, you enter your favourite restaurant, and it is busy. You know that your hearing health professional has set up programme two for just this very situation, so you switch your hearing aids to it.

You hear the two audible beeps, or if you are wearing a Widex it announces the programme name, and you know immediately you are at the right settings. It is still a bit loud though, so you turn down the volume a bit, the sound of the descending beeps let you know it is working. Simply put, audible indicators allow you confidence that you are using the hearing aid properly.

Listening programmes in hearing aids

Many hearing aid manufacturers offer listening programmes in their hearing aids. What they are is a differing number of pre-set listening situations that we can programme into hearing aids. Each listening programme has its settings optimised for different listening conditions/sound environments.

The different listening programmes can then be selected by the user using a switch or push button on the hearing instrument or via a remote control The listening conditions are usually set as speech, speech in noise, music and acoustic telephone.

What's the advantage to you?

Apart from the obvious one of offering better hearing in differing situations, there are other advantages. For instance, your hearing healthcare professional can make adjustments for just one situation in isolation without making global changes to how the hearing aids work.

That means that they can target changes to help you hear better in the situation you are having a problem with, without affecting the working of the hearing aids in other conditions where you are doing fine. In essence, the more programmes, the better the customisation of the hearing aid for you in different situations.

For a real-world instance, you leave the house in the morning with the children in the back of the car, so you change the listening programme to the one that focuses behind you so you can hear them clearly, all though in fairness after you did it, you wish you hadn't!.

After dropping them off you have to meet your friend in the coffee shop, the shop is busy so you use the programme that has been set up for noisy environments so you can hear her clearly. You are thrilled you did because she has some great news to share with you and you can hear it clearly. That is the benefit of listening programmes.

Automatic programmes in hearing aids

Many manufacturers offer different levels of automated programmes; what they do is automatically select the optimum instrument settings without the user having to push a button or use a switch. The management systems of the hearing instruments analyse and identify the current sound environment.

The management system decided what the best set of parameters for you to hear better in that sound situation and then automatically switches the parameters within the hearing aids to the appropriate settings. The amount of automatic programmes on any hearing aid is dependent on the manufacturer and the technology level.

What's the advantage to you?

Automatic programmes deliver real advantages; in essence, the hearing aids are always working to provide the best possible sound quality no matter where you are. They do so seamlessly and without any input from you, which means you can just concentrate on getting on with your life.

In most manufacturers' hearing aids, these automatic programmes can also be individually altered or fine-tuned for your preference. Most hearing aid manufacturers would also offer manual listening programmes alongside their automatic function. Again this delivers the benefit that your professional can provide the exact customised settings you need for just one situation.

Binaural synchronisation

Binaural synchronisation is something that has only recently entered the lexicon of hearing aid terms with the advent of wireless communication between hearing aids. In essence, it means that the hearing aids communicate wirelessly to ensure that the settings are synchronised.

What's the advantage to you?

Manufacturers introduced this hugely useful feature several years ago. At its most basic, this feature synchronises the current user settings across the two hearing aids. So if you make a change in one hearing aid, such as the changing the listening programme or volume control setting by touching the button, it is automatically switched on the other to reflect this. That means that the two devices are always in the same programme and at the same volume level.

However, it is at its most advanced where it dramatically improves the lives of hearing aid users. Binaural synchronisation, at its most sophisticated, makes sure that every feature of the hearing aid is working in a combined manner to deliver the very best listening experience.

That really is exciting stuff (god that was so geeky!) because it is responsible for the enormous advances in hearing aids in the last few years. It is also the reason why hearing aids have become more natural sounding (told you I was a nerd). When someone speaks about this technology to you, be sure to be clear precisely what it synchronises across the two hearing aids.

Binaural Compression

Again the advent of this feature was enabled because of the advances in wireless communication in hearing aids. Widex was first to introduce it in their flagship Clear hearing aids in 2009. Most of the manufacturers have followed suit in more recent times introducing the feature under differing names.

Hearing aids that use binaural compression work as a combined system to deliver enhanced sound as natural as possible. They achieve that by using both hearing aids to assess the surrounding sound environment. This information is then shared between and used by the hearing aids in a combined manner. This mass of information allows the hearing aids to make decisions on sound output as an actual pair or system.

What's the advantage to you?

The system uses natural sound cues such as temporal effects (time differences in sound) and the head shadow effect (differences in sound from one ear to the other) to assess what is going on in the sound environment. It then reproduces those sound cues in the enhanced sound you receive to deliver the most natural sound experience.

All of this happens instantaneously without time lag. Because they preserve the natural sound cues, your brain gets the optimum information possible so that it can do, what it does naturally. Remember, the ears just carry sound; it is the brain that makes sense of what you are hearing.

I think that this is the most exciting feature that has been released in recent times. As this feature evolves, it will make hearing aids better and better, achieving benefits for most users that were unimaginable even a few short years ago.

Compression channels

Compression channels have fallen out of favour recently as a sexy talked about feature because of two reasons. The first is that they are hard to explain without resorting to gobbledygook and the second being that sexier more understandable features have come about.

However, they are still fantastic features, and it is worth me trying to explain what they are. Okay, this is pretty technical stuff, but I will try to make it intelligible.

Compression channels are designed to change how different frequencies of sound are amplified. Compression channels are divided into several channels that are used to restrict or alter differing levels of amplification within one sound frequency.

For instance, you may have problems hearing sounds below 40dB in one channel. However, the amount of amplification we need to deliver to you to hear those sounds clearly is radically different from the amount of amplification that we may have to add to a sound of 65 dB. Compression channels allow us to add varying levels of amplification to the varying volume of sounds.

The feature is used to instruct the hearing aid to amplify or reduce the range of noises that you hear. This feature simply allows us to customise the hearing aids to your hearing loss in a better manner. Some hearing aids have more channels/bands than others.

What's the advantage to you?
Simply a better-customised hearing aid, which is the foundation that everything else relies upon.

Data logging

Data logging is a feature which records different sets of information during the hearing aid's use. Most hearing aid manufacturers offer data logging of one type or other with differing levels of data captured. This information is available to be analysed by the hearing professional when they connect to the hearing aids. This type of information allows a professional a deeper understanding of your experiences.

What's the advantage to you?
It can assist in the fine-tuning of the aid to your preferences. The data recorded includes the hours of use, the types of listening environments you were in, the listening programmes you used and any volume control changes during that period.

Data logging delivers information that helps the hearing professional to programme the hearing aid to your specific requirements. Anything that allows the programming of your hearing aids to better suit you has to be seen as a good thing.

Feedback cancellation in hearing aids

Feedback is the horrible whistling that is most associated with older hearing aids and used to be one of the biggest complaints of hearing aid users. Amplified sound being re-processed is what causes feedback, in other words, the sound emitted from the receiver (speaker) is re-processed through the hearing aids, and it shrieks. That is precisely the same thing that happens when you put a microphone too close to a speaker.

The underlying cause of the feedback is the escape of sound from the ear canal. There are many reasons for that; it can be due to poor fitting of an ear mould or in-ear hearing aid, which allows amplified sound to escape.

Earwax blockage is another frequent culprit for hearing aid feedback. Another cause of the feedback is the proximity of the hearing aids to something, for instance, if you place anything over your ear, a hand or hat or a person hugging you.

Feedback cancellation is a feature that identifies and stops feedback, how it does it changes from manufacturer to manufacturer and within technology levels. Suffice to say; each feature determines the feedback and the frequency or frequencies in which it is occurring.

It then removes the feedback from the signal and stops the whistling. Different features do this in different ways, I won't bore you with the technical details, but if you want to know, drop us a line, and we can explain.

What's the advantage to you?
Simply put, your hearing aid doesn't whistle, you don't get embarrassed, and your hearing aids work better.

Adaptive feedback cancellation

That is feedback cancellation on steroids, it can adapt its speed of operation to improve its performance automatically, and for example, it can change how it works when you are using a telephone, listening to music and suddenly hear alarm beeps.

The telephone needs strong feedback cancellation; the music situation needs very little feedback cancellation because musical notes can sound like feedback and alarm beeps is a similar concept.

Directional microphones

Directional microphones completely changed how hearing aid users can hear in noise. Directional microphone features use the sound information supplied by two microphones, to allow the computer brain of the hearing aid to identify the sound that is coming from the rear and sound that is coming from the front.

This allows the processor to reduce the level of sound coming from the rear and concentrate on the sound coming from the front. Modern directional microphone features enable you to change the direction of hearing as you require. You can change the focus of the hearing aids from all-around sound to being more focused on a single person or object to the front side or rear.

What's the advantage to you?
Simply put, directional microphones are a proven method for hearing well in noise. So they are an invaluable feature for you to have.

Adaptive directional microphones

Yes, you guessed it, directional microphones on steroids! This feature allows the null of the directional microphones to adapt; the null is where the noise source is. So the microphones detect the location of the loudest noise source and adjust the sound to reduce your perception of that noise.

If the noise source moves, the system adapts to keep that noise source reduced. Most of the modern adaptive systems work in more than one frequency band, meaning that they can help to reduce your perception of several different noises at one time, even if they are all moving to varying positions once they are at differing frequencies.

What is the advantage to you?
Bigger, better-proven method to help you hear in noisy environments!

Automatic directional microphones

That is a feature that just automates the directional microphones completely; it allows the processor to select how it will use the directional microphones according to the sound situation. In a quiet location, they will operate in an Omni-directional mode (taking in sound from all around) and directional mode or adaptive directional mode, if available, when a noise source is introduced.

What's the benefit to you?

Complete automation of what is an outstanding feature, you get to hear well in every situation without any input. It just happens automatically. Each manufacturer has its own flavour of directionality, where possible we will always explain what it is clearly on our website.

Frequency bands in hearing aids

Again, like compression bands or channels, this one is a little bit in-depth. Frequencies, as we will discuss them here, are the way that we split sound. Manufacturers divide the entire frequency range of a hearing instrument into several bands or channels in which we can customise the gain (amplification) to your hearing loss.

A quick but worthwhile side note here, the frequency bandwidth of hearing aids can be very different. What that means is that the number of sound frequencies that a hearing aid can process can be very different from manufacturer to manufacturer.

Some hearing aids can only process sound frequencies between 200 Hz and 6 kHz; others can handle between 100 Hz to 11.5 kHz. Why is this important? I hear you ask, while human speech is generally between 200 Hz and 4 to 6 kHz, for the full and rich enjoyment of music, a much wider bandwidth is more desirable.

Hence, if you are an audiophile, you might well appreciate the total bandwidth.

Back to frequency bands, each manufacturer is different; some hearing aid manufacturers call them bands and some call them channels, and some manufacturers offer more than others. The bands allow your professional to programme the hearing aid in a more customised way for your hearing loss. The more frequency bands that the hearing aid has, the finer the programme can be, so you end up with crisper, clearer hearing.

Most features of hearing aids work within the bands, so the more bands there are in the instrument, the more bands that the features in the hearing aid work across. How many bands are best? There is a lot of debate about that, but it is generally agreed that any amount between fifteen and twenty is optimal, that's why you will find most flagship hearing aids have numbers of channels or bands in that range.

For instance, Widex flagship hearing aids have fifteen channels. However, GN Resound hearing aids have seventeen channels.

What's the advantage to you?
The more frequency channels or bands hearing aids have, the better, although after twenty the benefit starts to fade. The more channels or bands, the better the customisation and the better experience that other hearing aid features will supply, which means that you will receive optimal benefit from your hearing aids.

Hearing aid noise reduction

That is probably the feature that drives most interest; it is often discussed as a feature that makes speech clearer in noise. Generally, it doesn't quite do that exactly. Only one manufacturer, Widex, has ever produced a noise reduction feature that affects the signal to noise ratio.

We use signal to noise ratio or SNR to geeks like me to measure the ratio of signal (speech) to noise. So the real measure of any feature that helps you to understand speech should be SNR. What most noise reduction features do is to reduce the amplification of non-speech sounds to allow a better understanding of speech sounds.

This tactic makes it more comfortable for a user in noisy conditions by reducing the background noise, for example in traffic noise in the street, a busy pub or restaurant. There is a lot of evidence that this reduces fatigue, reduces the amount of concentration you have to have and therefore, actually does help you hear speech a little clearer.

As with all features, not all noise reduction is the same, and the more high-end technology has better strategies to deal with noise.

What's the advantage for you?

A better chance for you to understand speech in noisier environments, in combination with a good directional microphone system it will dramatically improve your experience.

Speech enhancement

Speech enhancement is another feature designed to help you hear speech clearly in noise. It is used in combination with noise reduction to help you better understand those vital speech sounds. The processor in the hearing aids identifies speech signals and enhances or amplifies them. It analyses sound signals and, where most noisy maximises the speech signal.

What's the advantage for you?

In combination with noise reduction and directional microphones, it allows you the best opportunity to hear speech in noisy sound situations.

Transient noise reduction

That is simply a noise reduction feature that concentrates on identifying and suppressing impact or sudden sounds, such as shutting doors, clattering dishes and glass breaking. They design the feature to do it without affecting the speech clarity. It is known by many names across different hearing aid manufacturers.

No matter what they call it, it allows the hearing aid to process sudden or loud noises in a more comfortable way for the user.

What's the benefit for you?

A much more comfortable listening experience for you as you go about your daily life.

Wind noise reduction

It is what it sounds like; it is a noise reduction system that reduces the sound of wind cavitation on the hearing aid microphones. This feature is particularly useful for people who like to be in the outdoors. So if you are a golfer or a hiker, it is something that you should consider.

What's the benefit for you?
It will make it much easier for you to tolerate being outdoors if you are an outdoorsy type, golf and such things, it is an invaluable feature.

I think this covers the most apparent features available, as I said, different manufacturers call the features different things. But at their core, they are the features that I have discussed here. If I have missed something that you would like to know about, drop us a line on Hearing Aid Know, and we will answer your questions.

Over the Counter Hearing Aids

I spoke about this on Hearing Aid Know last year, but I think it is worth covering here. I believe that Over The Counter hearing aids will become a more significant feature of the hard of hearing world over the next few years. There has been growing speculation concerning Over the Counter (OTC) hearing aids being made legal in the United States, and finally in 2017, instructions were passed to the FDA to regulate for such devices.

The PCAST (PRESIDENT'S COUNCIL OF ADVISORS ON SCIENCE AND TECHNOLOGY) Report about hearing technology in October 2015 recommended a significant change to the laws governing the supply and provision of hearing aids. One of the recommendations it made was about the hearing aid medical waiver. That has now happened, what does it mean for OTC hearing aids and more importantly, what will it mean for consumers? Let's look at the background.

A Greedy Monopoly

For many years, hearing aid advocate organisations in the States have been calling for changes to the rules governing hearing aid provision. The main reason for these calls has been the assumption that the high price of hearing aids has been the main block to adoption of them by the multitude of people who need them. I don't necessarily subscribe to that argument; I know that cost is an issue for people; however, I don't feel it is the general impediment that it has been painted to be.

In this debate, both hearing aid manufacturers and providers of hearing aids, are painted as greedy and supporting a monopoly. Unfortunately, some of the hearing provider's representative organisations have not helped themselves with ridiculous paternalistic statements that seem to have been purposefully designed to irritate people.

Are We Greedy?

I know I am not; I would have to say the bulk of people who I know within the profession are not either. I charge for my time and service, and then I deliver that time and service as I am sure many others do. Focusing on the hearing aid as a product has not been helpful; it negates how that product is delivered and maintained. The problem though is that no matter what I say, it just looks like I am defending a monopoly.

On the 7th of December, the FDA issued the "Immediately in Effect Guidance Document: Conditions for Sale for Air-

Conduction Hearing Aids," which effectively ends federal enforcement of the hearing aid medical waiver. What does that mean for the consumer? The hearing aid medical waiver is a waiver that may be signed instead of having the required pre-hearing-aid-purchase medical evaluation.

The wording of the federal regulation can be seen here (21CFR801.421). In essence, it removes the need for a customer over the age of eighteen to get a medical evaluation of their hearing before deciding on hearing aids.

The FDA announcement does not change any rules regarding over-the-counter (OTC) hearing aids, but it did address them. "FDA does intend to consider and address those recommendations in the future as appropriate, including those regarding a regulatory framework for hearing aids that can be sold directly to consumers, without the requirement for consultation with a credentialed dispenser. FDA intends to solicit additional public input from stakeholders before adopting such an approach".

In the press release " the FDA Commissioner Robert Califf, M.D. was quoted as saying "Today's actions are an example of the FDA considering flexible approaches to regulation that encourage innovation in areas of rapid scientific progress, The guidance will support consumer access to most hearing aids while the FDA takes the steps necessary to propose to modify our regulations to create a category of OTC hearing aids that could help many Americans improve their quality of life through better hearing." I think that was taken as a clear sign that with time, OTC hearing aids will become a reality.

For many years I have spoken with hearing aid advocates around the world, advocates like Steve my co-author Hearing Aid Know. Nearly all of them have been demanding more power over their hearing aids, the ability to make fine-tuning changes themselves. I have always supported that idea: why shouldn't we make their hearing care inclusive?

One thing that has always struck me during these conversations is that what they called for was the inclusion in the process, not the exclusion of the professional. Even the most strident and independent of Advocates want the ability to consult with an expert.

Would it surprise you to find out that I would support this type of hearing devices? Because I would.

You may find it surprising, but I think these types of devices are a good thing, not a bad thing. However, they will only be a good thing if we can meet specific criteria. You will need to be able to fit the devices to your loss in some way. There needs to be some way of testing your needs either built into the device or accompanying it. Any testing procedure needs to be able to flag referable conditions; this is imperative.

In my career, I have identified four people with cancer through a hearing test. I, of course, did not make that diagnosis; I simply undertook the hearing test and referred them for further investigation because I was deeply unhappy with the results— four people who went on to have lifesaving treatment because of a hearing test.

Hearing loss is more often than not run of the mill hearing loss; however, sometimes it is not. Sometimes it is a sign of some underlying nefarious condition that needs treatment. That is what scares other people and me within the profession. However, good technology can probably ensure that it is not an issue. I think it is incumbent upon the FDA and any other regulatory body to provide some sort of strong regulations are in place concerning this.

What will it Mean For You

When they bring the new legislation forward to legalise the sale of OTC hearing aids, it will mean that you can go to your local point of sale and buy an OTC hearing aid just like you would purchase any electronic device. You will then have to work out how to fit it and use it flying solo as it were. I think that this type of solution will not be a fit for everyone, and I don't believe the devices will be any better than very basic hearing aids.

Not for Everyone

Even within the traditional hearing aid manufacturers, there has been a push towards giving users more control over the hearing devices. However, some users aren't interested in having the power; in fact, many want something that they put on and never have to think about again.

OTC devices will be ideal for some and not for others. There was a recent small-scale study on the efficacy of self-fitted hearing aids that I reported on. The conclusions were fascinating, although the study was small, it has added some weight to the call for further research. Its findings were as follows

"While limited, the data suggest that self-fitting aids may provide satisfactory benefit and performance to those who can manage the self-fitting process. Our findings show that at least one currently available self-fitting product is comparable to those measured with professionally dispensed hearing aids."

What they said, in essence, was that when people were "able to manage" it seemed that self-fitting might not be a bad thing. By able to manage, they meant technically aware and capable, people who were au fait or familiar with the technology.

In this context, I think that OTC hearing aids will be very similar; they will be ideal for people who can manage them. However, they might not be suitable for everyone. I believe they will be similar in concept to many of the hearing aids available now as internet sales.

The Freedom to Mess it up

These devices will also give you the freedom to make a mess of your hearing; this is another factor that the FDA needs to consider. It needs to ensure that you can't make your hearing worse through the use of these devices. Again, I think technology can help here, but it is an issue that we must raise. In essence, for these devices to be safe to use, users will need some education about making them safe to use.

I have talked to others within the business for some time about adopting low-cost devices that were sold on an over the counter type basis. I would adopt these types of devices; I would insist that I did a workup on your hearing or you had a workup done by someone I trust (this is to protect both you and me). I would then sell you the device for you to do with it what you wanted.

If you want support or help other than a warranty issue, I will charge you for it. I think that is fair; my time is worth money, you would not expect to attend any other professional for consultation for free, so why would you expect to do so with me? I think that this may well be the future model; I don't think the traditional model will die quite yet. I believe this new model will probably run in tandem with the conventional model.

What about Traditional Manufacturers?

What will the traditional hearing aid manufacturers do when OTC comes to pass? I don't know, I can't speak for them, but I think they will have to re-assess their ideas about provision channels. I don't and would not hold that against them; it is just the way of the world and business.

As I mentioned earlier, Sonova purchased Blamey Saunders, an online hearing device retailer in Australia in 2019. They then introduced Shift Hearing in conjunction with Blamey Saunders. Shift hearing aids are self-fit hearing devices using the same technology that underpins Phonak Marvel hearing aids.

They offer the hearing aids with ongoing support if needed, which is provided by the Blamey Saunders team. In essence, this is a blended model owned by a significant mainstream hearing device manufacturer. While it remains to be seen whether it is successful, I feel that it will probably serve as a template for the other hearing aid manufacturers moving forward.

I know that many manufacturers wouldn't be eager to become involved in the OTC market. However, business is like an arms race, when one-ups the game, the others must do so to survive. As well as that, many of the hearing aid manufacturers are public companies; their management teams will need to make decisions based on their shareholders best interests.

It would be my feeling that they will take a watching brief on the market and then decide to enter it.

What Will Be Your Experience?

I think that depends on who makes the devices, hearing aids are a specialist electronic device. Hearing aid manufacturers are producing useful devices based on years of experience and research and design. New entrants to the market don't necessarily have that experience or the algorithms that make everything work.

A hearing aid is not just a simple amplifier; it does so much more than amplify sound. So it will be interesting to see what the first OTC hearing aids are like. If traditional manufacturers become involved in this market and follow the Shift Hearing template, it will mean that there will be some pretty good devices available.

Care of the Devices

Any buyer of these devices will have to take care of them, and any vendor will have to consider the failure of the receiver. It is pretty simple, earwax and moisture kill receivers (the speaker part) and any seller of the devices will have to be aware of that.

At the moment, traditional hearing aid manufacturers accept when your negligence (and that is often what it is) kills one of their receivers during the warranty period. They simply replace them, even when they are gummed up with ear wax.

How will that work with over the counter hearing aids? Will they continue to replace the receiver even when you have been responsible for its failure? I mean at the moment, the hearing aid manufacturers don't have to, but they do it. What will OTC manufacturers do?

Making the Right Choice

I try to be very careful about the recommendation I make; I try to take into account lifestyle, personal and ear canal conditions. For instance, if you are active, able, and a bit tech-smart, I will easily consider a RIC device or a custom hearing aid device for you. I would base that on the fact that you can easily take care of the device, ensuring that it is maintained so that the receiver won't fail.

If however, I think that the maintenance of the hearing aid may be a problem, or if in fact, the ear canal is just too hostile (excess ear wax or moisture) I would nearly always recommend a BTE. As a purchaser of OTC devices, how will you make the decision on that? If you make the wrong decision, what are you going to do?

Freedom

It is evident that there are a lot of questions to answer, however I think that OTC hearing aids will bring freedom of choice. I think that can be a good thing and a bad thing. I don't think consumers are stupid, generally, well most of them. I believe that delivering freedom of choice will allow people to adopt amplification earlier. Will enable them to test the water as it were, to understand what amplification can provide to their life. That has to be a good thing.

Clean and Care of Hearing Aids

Hearing aids are small, electronic devices that operate in conditions that are both warm and damp. Conditions that most electronics don't like. After making a significant investment in being able to hear better, it makes a lot of sense for you to keep them in the best shape possible by cleaning and maintaining them at home.

The hearing aid manufacturers make great efforts to ensure your hearing aid will keep on keeping on. However, if you don't do your part, those hearing aids will fail. In many cases, a failure may well end up needing to be sent away for repair.

That could leave you without your hearing aid for up to two weeks, depending on how busy the repair centres are. That is a significant hassle; in my experience, people who have become used to better hearing with their hearing aids hate to be without them. It upsets them, so the key is to maintain your hearing aids as much as possible to avoid any hassle.

Avoid hearing aid repairs

Hearing aids do fail, it is a fact of life, electronic components can fail, and they certainly will with age and constant use. But you can take steps to avoid that failure for as long as possible. You should incorporate those step into a good daily clean and care routine.

Most of the time, I was in Practice, the failures I saw were a receiver (loudspeaker part) or microphone failures. It was exceptionally rare to see anything else within a hearing aid fail. Both of these components are the most exposed in every hearing aid.

They are the components that need daily attention. Some hearing aid types are more prone to possible failure than others. For instance, in the ear hearing aids and receiver in the canal hearing aids have a higher failure rate than behind the ear hearing aids.

Hearing Aid Care and Maintenance

So let's get to the meat, how you can best take care of your aids, I will discuss each type of aid, and each step that you need to take. If I miss anything, let me know. Likewise, if you have some excellent tips yourself, don't hesitate to contact us. Before we move on here is some quick tips for hearing aid nirvana:

Follow a daily routine

Clean the hearing aids giving attention to the receivers and microphones

Dry out your hearing aids

Quick tip:

Never use alcohol, solvents or cleaning agents on your hearing aids. Special care products for cleaning like hearing aid wipes and sprays are available, and you should use them.

Cleaning of hearing aids and cleaning tools

You should clean your hearing aid every day; every manufacturer supplies a cleaning kit with their hearing aids.

It will usually include a wax brush, a wax pick and a cloth. Manufacturers design these tools to help you care for your aids and using them properly will help to keep your hearing aids going.

Hearing aid manufacturers have also designed filters to protect receivers in the case of RIC and ITE hearing aids.

You will also get at least one pack of these with your hearing aids. **Use Them,** the proper use of wax filters (sometimes called wax caps) will protect your receiver and keep it going longer.

Quick Tip:

Earwax & moisture kills hearing aids; wax guards are there for a reason, use them!

The most significant cause of failure is wax and moisture getting into the receivers or the microphones of hearing aids. If you change your wax guards when you should, you can avoid much of this problem.

When do wax guards need to be changed?

I am sorry, but the honest answer is how long is a piece of string? Each person is different; I have seen Patients who only needed to replace their wax guards once every six months, I have seen other Patients that needed to change them every month.

It depends on wax production in the ear canal. Generally, as a rule of thumb, if your wax guard is full of wax that doesn't fall out when brushed, it is time to replace it. If you don't, that wax will eventually make it into the sound tube and then the receiver.

Cleaning and maintenance of an ITE and RIC hearing aid

ITE hearing aids, in particular, need daily attention, as do RIC hearing aids. The reason for this is that the receiver lives in the ear in both devices. As I said earlier, these devices are equipped with wax guards of which you need to pay special attention. So let's break down the steps you need to take and when you should take them:

Quick tip:

Many people try to clean their aid at the end of the day; I always recommended doing it in the morning after drying it overnight. That way the wax is dry and easier to remove.

1. Place your hearing aids in a drying device at the end of the day. That will allow the removal of moisture from both the electronics and any wax or debris gathered on the aid.
2. The next morning, have a good look at the microphone inlets and the receiver end of the hearing aids. Get yourself a magnifying glass if you need to for this. The details and placement of these areas will be in your owner's manual or your hearing professional will show you.

3.   Concentrate on cleaning the receiver and microphone ports using the soft-bristle brush that came with the cleaning kit. When you do it in the morning, the wax should be dried out and easy to move, especially after drying out overnight.

4.   To clean off built-up wax, hold the hearing aid and gently clean the openings with the wax brush. The dried debris should be loose enough to be cleaned away.

5.   If there is still wax in the ports that have not been dislodged, you can use your wax pick (again, usually included in your cleaning kit) to clear more stubborn deposits out of the ports. Be careful here, don't jab the pick in, just use it gently.

6.   Check your battery compartment and the battery contacts for wax or debris, if there is any brush it off.

7.   Finish by wiping the entire hearing aid with the cloth provided. That will remove leftover debris from the hearing aid.

8.   Assess your wax guard, if it looks like it needs changing, change it. If you change your wax guard when needed, it will go a long way towards reducing failures.

9.   Lastly, give your hearing aids a good visual once-over, with ITEs, check the casing and any joins for any signs of cracks or issues. With RIC devices check the receiver wire, make sure there are no kinks or twists that may lead to the failure of the wire.

Cleaning & Maintenance of BTE hearing aids

BTE hearing aids are much harder to kill. However, you still need to clean and maintain them. Drying them is as essential as it is for ITE and RIC aids. The maintenance is similar but different. So let's break down the steps you need to take and when you should take them:

Quick tip:

Drying is as vital for BTEs as any other hearing aid, especially the tubes.

1. Place your hearing aids in a drying device at the end of the day, that will allow moisture to be removed from both the electronics and any wax or debris gathered on the aid.

2. Occasionally when needed, remove the ear mould and tube (if you have one) from the hook and clean it with soapy water. If your BTE has a thin tube, remove the thin tube and use the supplied wire (like a hair-thin pipe cleaner) to push through the tube. That will remove any debris.

3. Use an air blower to force water out of the tube and then place the tubing in the drying kit with your hearing aid to dry overnight.

4. The next morning, have a good look at the microphone inlets of the hearing aids. Again a magnifying glass can be helpful. The details and placement of these areas will be in your owner's manual or your hearing professional will show you.

5. Concentrate on cleaning around the microphone ports and any other user controls like programme buttons or volume controls. Use the soft-bristle brush that came with the cleaning kit. Again, doing this in the

morning is the ideal time, the wax should be dried out and easy to move, especially after drying out overnight.

6. To clean off built-up wax, hold the hearing aid and gently clean it with the wax brush. The dried debris should be loose enough to clean away.

7. If there is still wax in the ports that haven't dislodged, you can use your wax pick (again, usually included in your cleaning kit) to clear more stubborn deposits. Be careful here, don't jab the pick in, just use it gently.

8. Check your battery compartment and the battery contacts for wax or debris, if there is any brush it off.

9. Finish by wiping the entire hearing aid with the cloth provided. That will remove leftover debris from the hearing aids.

10. Lastly, give your hearing aids a good visual once-over, check the casing and any joins for any signs of cracks or issues.

Drying out hearing aids

I have spoken several times about drying out your hearing aids in this section; I should explain the process and what you can use to do it.

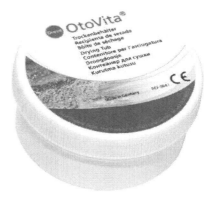

Hearing aid dryers

Hearing aid drying equipment comes in all shapes and sizes

from the very cheap to moderately expensive.

It is one of the single most important investments you will make if you buy a hearing aid. Moisture build-up in hearing aids cause real issues and failures, and it is generally easy to avoid.

Hearing aid drying cups and tablets

Probably the most straightforward and cheapest form of hearing aid drying available but still very effective. It is merely a jar/cup with a sealable lid to which you drop a drying tablet. Every night you screw the lid off, drop your hearing aids in and seal it.

The tablets are designed to suck moisture out of the air and your hearing aids. In the morning, take your hearing aids out (don't forget to seal the lid again) and voila, dry hearing aids. It is a simple process, easy to do and will save you real money in repair costs, so why wouldn't you do it?

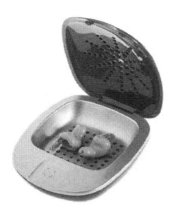

Electronic hearing aid dryers

Yes, you guessed it, hearing aid dryers you plug in. They come with different functionality, some will still use drying tablets or bricks, and some don't. Some will dry your hearing aids and disinfect them using UV light; some won't. Many of them are designed to be portable so that you can bring them with you on trips.

Widex introduced a drying station late last year; they call it the Dry N Go. It is a portable electronic drying and disinfecting station. There are several available on the market though.

If you follow a good clean and care routine, your hearing aids will function better for longer. Hearing aid repairs are expensive enough, so take care to avoid them with some simple maintenance.

In Finishing

I like helping people; it is one of my things. Don't think this is just some selfless, altruistic streak. There is some of that involved, but I get a buzz knowing I helped someone. So it isn't precisely unselfish.

I would ask you to do me a great favour; if you have found this book to be of real use to you, I would ask you to give it a favourable review where you have bought it. Your reviews are valuable; they provide the next person looking for information the confidence to buy the book.

I have covered much here, and I hope I have made it clear and easy to read, however, if I have not, or if you are looking for more information, don't hesitate to contact us with your questions on Hearing Aid Know.

Printed in Great Britain
by Amazon